An Alzheimer's Journey: Carolyn's Return to Birth

EDWARD ALDERETTE

An Alzheimer's Journey: Carolyn's Return to Birth

DEDICATION

To Carolyn Alderette

and all who loved her, especially those
who helped care for her in her return to birth.

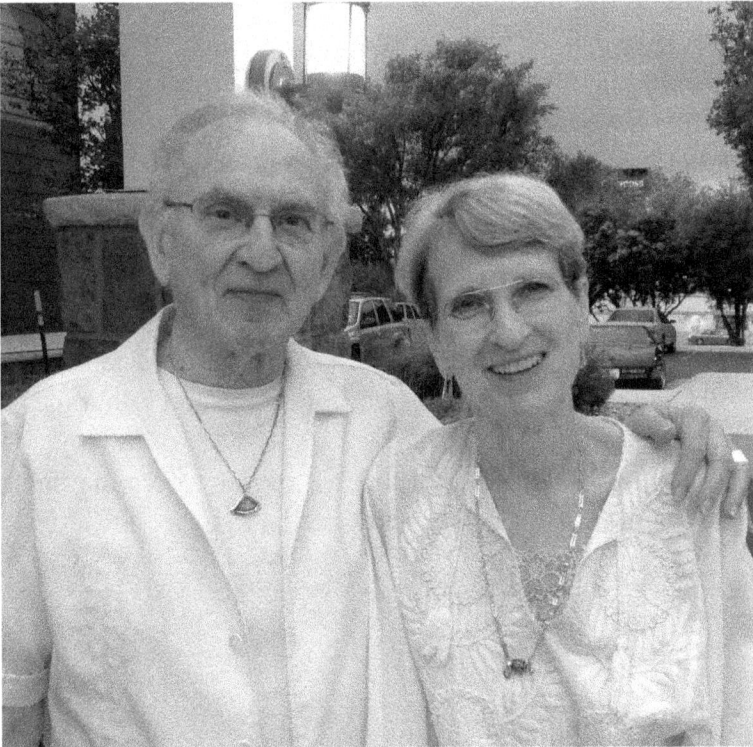

Edward and Carolyn Alderette in April of 2013

ACKNOWLEDGEMENTS

I acknowledge the incredible service of Mireya Hinojosa (a nursing student at the time) for the patience in transcribing the first draft from my hand-printed manuscript. (Handwritten, printed hand scratching is still hand scratching, just like the proverbial monkey-in-silks is still a monkey.) Mireya went on to do two more typed drafts of edited works before I handed the typed manuscript to my niece, Eileen.

To Eileen, I owe the acknowledgement of having taken that copy in order to rearrange it to the specifications for publication. She did more than that. She did the work of a literary agent, procuring an ISBN and managing the elements of design and printing.

These two women, whom I thank profusely, were the richest hands-on support I had for getting out Carolyn's story.

INTRODUCTION

This story centers around Carolyn. It entails sadness of the most profound... and like many of life's stories about normal people, this one witnesses many experiences along the way which were fraught with the dark side of life. Despite this pain and suffering, there appeared events of good and of consummate value, if not in every everyday, frequently enough for honest to goodness hope to rise from the ashes of that dark side.

I choose to open this story with Carolyn's obituary. This serves to present a thumbnail, thimble-full sketch of what Carolyn (Sara Carolyn Knott Alderette) had made of herself before Alzheimer's disease took her to retrogenesis.

The ultimate of retrogenesis is death. Retrogenesis means return to birth.

No matter how incrementally it travels, this process culminates in death. (As of this writing medical science does not have the answer for arresting the disease).

This story highlights how Alzheimer's went down its inexorable path in the case of Carolyn and, by association, of Edward, me, her primary caregiver for the duration of the journey.

Edward Alderette

CHAPTER ONE
THE MOMENT IN A NUTSHELL

Obituary for Sara Carolyn Alderette
April 26, 1943- June 6, 2015
Published in the San Antonio Express-News on June 9, 2015

Carolyn Alderette, the former Sara Carolyn Knott, born to Sara Jim Hilley and Kenneth L. Knott of Dallas, TX, April 26, 1943, died on June 6, 2015.

She graduated in 1961 as Valedictorian from Berlin High School in Germany where her mother and step-father Lt. Col. Harry G. Sherblom were stationed after World War II.

In 1965 she graduated from UTEP, then known as Texas Western College of Mines in El Paso, TX, as Outstanding Senior and with the Golden Scroll of Scholastic Achievement. She was a member of Zeta Tau Alpha Sorority.

In 1968 she and Edward Alderette of El Paso, TX, were married in New Orleans, LA, where they would both eventually complete Masters Degrees at Tulane University School of Social Work.

She developed a great and accomplished talent of renovating old houses which she put to use for personal historic homes in Lexington, KY (1973-1975), Atlanta, GA (1975-1977), and in the King William Historic District of San Antonio, TX (1977-1981).

The avocation of home restoration and her study of accounting and bookkeeping practices while in Atlanta, GA, at Georgia State University, led her to pursue courses in blueprint reading at Our Lady of the Lake University in San Antonio, TX, and to work for a local renovation constructing company, Winn Construction, as Office Manager (1978-1981).

From 1981 to 1983, she was employed by Finidam Assistant Building Manager of Place St. Charles, a high-rise building in downtown New Orleans, LA.

In 1983, Edward took a position as a psychotherapist with the offices of Harry Croft and Associates, in San Antonio, TX, and Carolyn became a Medical Social Worker at Methodist Hospital. She did Home Health Social Work and became the Director of Family Friends under the aegis of Any Baby Can. From 1997 until her retirement in 2007, she was the Director of Admissions for Morningside Ministries on Babcock Road.

After retirement, she worked approximately three years as a volunteer at Morningside Ministries Gift Shop, just to stay close to the geriatric people whom she loved to serve.

Her love for working with Senior Citizens extended to aiding their family and friends. Her devotion to this work led her to excel in the labyrinthical rules and regulations of Medicare and Medicaid so that she could navigate families to needed resources for loved ones.

Wherever Carolyn worked and whatever she did, she maintained a record of "Summa Cum Laude" evaluations for the quantity and quality and the theory and practice which she exhibited in her professional performance.

Carolyn beat cancer twice; once, through a courageous total hysterectomy and, again, through a lumpectomy.

Not being able to grace life's garden with progeny of her own was a tough regret to overcome; showering love on her younger sisters and multiple nieces and nephews, especially Eileen and Emily the daughters of the brother she cherished, helped her to bear 'no child of her own.'

Family, especially her early and hearty ties to the two Kens in her life, her dad and her brother, founded her in firm convictions about where love truly begins. From there she went to palpable compassion for the poor and the unprotected, including those in the animal kingdom. Her favorite charities were for those populations.

Carolyn believed in understated elegance in fashion and dressed accordingly; that gene she inherited from her mother.

Her artistic eye for home decoration and color, especially her predilections for Southwest art, was strictly of her divination.

One maternal aunt gave to her and to her brother a penetrating appreciation and vocabulary for living creatures of all sizes: from the sweeping hawk to the purring kitty and from the massive cats to the horny toad.

That same aunt instilled in young Carolyn and Ken the vision to see Spirit permeating all such life. In adulthood, Carolyn came to recognize that self-same Spirit in "the solidity of the mountain" and the "flexibility of the wind" and in all created beings. From there emerged her all-encompassing theology: there is Spirit in everything and every one and that Spirit is the Creator, all One, and, of course, to her that is the end and the beginning of the Mystery.

The finesse in nurturance and display of affection which she readily displayed to family and others, alike, she inherited from another maternal aunt.

Carolyn was preceded in death by her dad and stepmother, Kenneth and Janie Knott; by her mom and stepfather, Sara and Harry Sherblom; by her brother Ken Knott of Montgomery, AL, as well as all paternal and maternal grandparents and all aunts and uncles.

If Carolyn would have contributed to her own obituary, she probably would have added: "Creator, you have given us tough and even more magnificent life. Thank you, Creator."

Survivors include: Edward Alderette, her husband of 47 years and her sisters: Sue Ellen Sherblom (G. Thomas Woodard) of Arnold, MD, and Lisa Sherblom of San Antonio, TX, and multiple nieces and nephews and grand nieces and nephews.

CHAPTER TWO
THE NEWNESS OF THE MOMENT

I invite you, just for a moment, to allow yourself to imagine that you are about to sit down to an ordinary dinner on an ordinary Saturday ("as the world turns").

Imagine that you are in your kitchen, in a home which you and your spouse have occupied for 28 years, and you are with a person whom you have lived with and loved for 44 years as your spouse.

Imagine, in your next breath, that your spouse has just sat down next to you where you have been waiting, sitting, beginning to start eating, and that she sits herself down and looks at you sideways for just a moment and quietly, with no alarm in her voice, asks you: "Who are you? What's your name?"

Imagine that her questions - strange questions to you coming from your spouse of 44 years of marriage - are rooted in her experienced perception that you are a total stranger at her table and she does not know who you are nor what you are doing there.

Next in this imaginary scenario see that she suddenly realizes, "…and, oh! My husband is not here." She is not remembering that the "you" sitting there is the husband she is missing. She just now realized: "He's not here and he ought to be here." It's taking her a while to realize that, not only is her husband missing, she is conversing with a perfect stranger whom she is treating as if they were meeting in some restaurant. She has a "perfect" recollection of her husband but the "you" sitting there is not him.

This is precisely how Alzheimer's disease introduced itself into Carolyn's and my world. It was an ordinary dinner time when the 69-year-old Carolyn and the 78-year-old Edward, me, living the middle-class life of two retired professionals - MSW's both from Tulane - sat down for what turned out to be the most unordinary dinner of their entire life.

She actually looked at me sideways as she sat next to me and quietly (with no alarm in her voice) asked: "Who are you?" and "What is your name?"

She is asking me as if I am a total stranger, and, no, we are not at some restaurant and meeting by happenstance. We are sitting at our kitchen table, and, all of a sudden, our entire lives are being upended as if our history together never happened. She is acting with me as if we never had a history together. Not only is there "no alarm in her voice," there is no animosity, no sign of having forgotten my name. She knew the name of her husband Edward; she also knew this was a total stranger in her kitchen, not Edward.

At first, her mood takes the path of quizzicalness as to who might I be and what might I be doing there.

The alarm going off silently but screamingly inside of my halted heartbeat, my challenged psyche, my struggling equilibrium, and my totally confused ego, revolved around how to interpret what confronted me when her doubts as to who I was confronted me.

My immediate past as an active psychotherapist for 31 years sounded those alarms which I needed to face. In those 31 years I saw, more than once, the whole gamut of mental health dysfunction from the simple neurosis to the extreme psychosis. The entire spectrum from "just" nervous to "insane-out-of-touch-with-reality-and-in-need-of-psychiatric-confinement" had been the realities of patients in my care.

On that May 12, 2012, I knew that I witnessed and did not imagine that in one fell swoop my wife was not in touch with reality.

Where did she lose the ability to recognize me as the person whom I have been for the last 44 years of her life? The answer was: right there in that kitchen that night, without any fanfare, she lost the ability to recognize me, and I could not believe what I was believing despite years of experience with psychiatric problems - 31 to be exact.

Partly because I had worked extensively and intensively with post-traumatic stress disorder, I had also studied and rehearsed how not to allow a major crisis to throw one into PTSD, i.e., paralysis of the mind. I engaged in what athletes and warriors engage in, staying centered so as to be able to go to centeredness even in the presence of a major turbulence.

So, I responded to her in my (controlled) quietest voice, "Carolyn, I am Ed." She answered: "How do you know my name? I don't know who you are." She still hadn't averted to the absence of her husband. Again, I stuck to the rational approach: "I am Ed; I am Edward." She said, "I've been married to Edward a long time. You are not him. By the way, where is Edward? Where did he go? Why isn't he here?"

As she calmly (as in not hurting) asks this and her questions multiply, I am wondering apprehensively how far does this go? I wonder if I need to be prepared for violence from her since my answer is not satisfying her as I am wondering where does this stop? I am increasingly aware that nothing in my background has equipped me to make this situation we are both in better, yet I am managing to stay centered.

So I sit in stunned disbelief, waiting for this reality - this circumstance - to change, waiting for her to snap back into my reality just as quickly and as simply as she snapped out of it. Nothing changed. From that Saturday night until four days later, Wednesday, we went over the same territory repeatedly. In that period of time she asked me to prove what was to her my ridiculous assertion that I was her husband Edward and, when I showed her my driver's license, she immediately recognized my wallet as Edward's and wanted to know how I had gotten it. She knew the wallet was his because she had given it to him. This, of course, was true; she had bought it for me in Buenos Aires.

The picture of me on my driver's license incensed her because she knew that was Edward's picture. She could look at the picture and see Edward but her "condition" prevented her from seeing me as the same person as the one on that driver's license. What incensed her was that for me to have "his" valuables meant I had to have taken them from "him."

In those initial days she saw me wearing Edward's clothes and his jewelry, and her worry increased that I might have injured Edward to acquire "his" possessions. I witnessed her recognizing some things which belonged to our shared reality but not my face from that reality. My clothes? Yes. My jewelry? Yes. My driver's license? Yes. "When," I kept wondering, "will she recognize my face? As Edward's?"

Nothing in her demeanor indicated that would happen.

We were both very confused and for two very different reasons. Her confusion was scaring her. She was 100% convinced she was dealing with a stranger. She was not confused about herself; she was confused about him - the one who was insisting that he was her husband.

18

In those initial days my awareness grew and made me more than quite grateful to the Creator that nothing of violence had transpired. She had grabbed at my wallet, and I let her have it versus playing tug-of-war with her. Later, I just took it from where she had laid it down.

There was no threatened violence to herself or to the house. Many years prior I had personally been called at 11:30 p.m. to the home of one of my former patients who had lost touch with the reality which we are in. This former patient was in the process of destroying every single piece of stoneware of a 60-piece set in the home he shared with with his family and threatening violence to anyone who tried to stop him. He had to reduce every piece in their kitchen to smithereens before he allowed me to talk him into going that very night to a psychiatric unit.

I was most grateful that nothing like that was happening in our house of 28 years. Grateful, yes, a hundred times over, but also apprehensive that something violent might/could erupt at any minute. I simply did not know.

In those initial days it would dawn on her over and over again that if I were in possession of Edward's things I must have taken them from him. Then she would panic, thinking that I had (must have) done harm to her husband.

"Did you kill him?"
"Where did he go, then, without his possessions?"
"And without telling me where he was going?"

In order to disarm the alarm going on in her confused state, I assured her more than once that none of the possessions which she was seeing on me would ever leave this house and that she would be constantly seeing them. I also repeatedly tried to reassure her that, no, I had definitely not harmed her husband nor anyone else.

It later dawned on me how defensive I had felt just being regarded as a killer.

These types of assurances delivered quietly (and not defensively) definitely helped her feel like she was exerting some control over some of the chaos in her perception.

CHAPTER THREE
THE UNFOLDING OF THE MOMENT

Between that fateful Saturday and the following Wednesday I contacted her closest relatives to tell them how I was a total stranger to Carolyn and that I knew not why. I was hoping against hope that we would soon be in the presence of Lisa, Carolyn's one sister in town, so that her sister's recognition of me as the Edward she was seeking would somehow trigger off some mechanism in Carolyn's mind and help her to see the same Edward. When the three of us did meet, Carolyn continued seeing "the stranger" regardless of what her sister saw.

One relative, Carolyn's sister-in-law and a widow since Carolyn's brother's death in 2007, drove 900 miles from Titus, Alabama, to our home in San Antonio as soon as she was appraised of the situation. In the meantime, Carolyn had herself called Lisa and relatives in Alabama to tell them of the stranger in her house who was not going away. She had called some women friends in town also, telling them she was scared this man might harm her. She never indicated to me that she felt she was in danger from me.

She talked by phone to a nephew-in-law of ours, telling him of her predicament, and he asked her if that stranger was with her as they talked. When she answered in the affirmative, he asked her to allow him to talk to me, the stranger. Carolyn agreed. I talked briefly with our nephew, and, when Carolyn took the phone again, he told her that he could tell that "that man" was not dangerous and he was not going to hurt her and that she could trust him.

The nephew vouched for me and she was able to trust the trust he conveyed. Small occurrences like this felt like tremendous victories amidst an ocean of uncertainties.

For two months we did not know Carolyn's diagnosis. I had begun channeling hand-delivered letters to her primary physician two days prior to her scheduled visits. The letter would detail for the doctor what Carolyn's symptoms were and descriptions of her behavior so that the doctor would not be surprised at the time of the visit.

That physician quite adroitly took the given information plus her own observations of Carolyn's behaviors and, with great compassion, convinced Carolyn to have MRI's, PET scans, plus newly established relations with a highly reputable neurologist and psychiatrist to work on cognitive dysfunction. Prior to the May 12, 2012, incident, Carolyn had been telling her primary of her great concern with "dropping words." Carolyn was forgetting multiple things including the ability to recall certain words. Her primary persuaded Carolyn that this was a light case of cognitive dysfunction.

In July of 2012, we received neurological testing results confirming a pattern consistent with Alzheimer's disease. The PET scan revealing these results guided Carolyn's neurologist and psychiatrists until they were able to administer their own testing. Within two months of the original episode of May 12, 2012, Carolyn's three physicians, primary, neurologist, and psychiatrist, were all in agreement that she was on the road of Alzheimer's. Carolyn heard the diagnosis one time from a nurse practitioner but did not believe it.

My observation and that of the people around her did not require a name, a classification, or a diagnosis to see that the patient, the woman not knowing her husband, the woman who had been having more and more cognitive dysfunction in forgetfulness of words and inability to finish a sentence and a harder and harder time dealing with the concept of time and calendar, was suffering tremendously. I could see it more because I was around her 24/7. I heard the fears behind: "Where is my husband?" "Did he abandon me?" "Is he dead?" "Will this stranger hurt me?" "Did he hurt my husband?" "Was my husband kidnapped?" "Will I be?" "Can anyone help me?" "Will Edward return?"

My situation constituted a tremendous stressor, just from the viewpoint of not having a ready answer for all these "logical" questions of Carolyn's. Nothing I ventured quelled her anxiety. There was nothing I could do to alter the trajectory of our life. I can honestly report that from May 12, 2012, to June 6, 2015, I constantly worked to stay super alert to prevent every unknown new situation from taking me to the heights of panic and/or anxiety attacks or to its companion depression. I suffered horrendous pain emotionally, but the Conscious Universe enabled me to avoid major depression and anxiety attacks. To suffer those mental states is pathological, to experience grief is not.

I could see that my wife suffered even more stress and anxiety because her condition precluded any ability to de-stress herself from the fears indicated by the questions she asked and for which no one around could give her satisfactory answers. I witnessed first-hand how erroneous the oft-quoted thing about Alzheimer's is - the one that pronounces: "The Alzheimer's patient does not suffer," (the implied reason being, he/she is not in touch with the real). The pronouncement goes on to say: "It is the attending caregiver(s) who suffer(s)."

As a caregiver, I suffered exceedingly and to the point of painful tears, but the burn of the tears became more pronounced as I witnessed the crucible of suffering Carolyn experienced in crying out the questions for which no one could give a satisfactory answer.

From her psychiatrist, we obtained written information about the syndrome accounting for her inability to recognize me as her husband. The syndrome is called Capgras, taken from the French name of the doctor who first described its sometimes existence in the patient on the road to Alzheimer's.

I believe that, just as it was intended to be a help to begin this saga with Carolyn's obituary, it will also be of extreme clarification to give a descriptive definition here of Alzheimer's disease. I want to present a chart outlining seven major gradations to which a patient declines in the progression of this disease: Alzheimer's.[1]

---

[1] Sharon L. Lewis, *Stress-Busting Program for Family Caregivers: A Path to Wellness,* (San Antonio: University of Texas Health Science Center, 2008), 51.

Retrogenesis (Back to Birth)

Stage	Alzheimer's Disease-Related Dementias (ADRD)	Stage*	Developmental Age*	Diversion/Distraction Activities
Mild	No difficulty at all	1		
	Some memory trouble begins to affect job/home. Forgets familiar names.	2		
	Much difficulty maintaining job performance. Withdrawal from difficult situations.	3	12+ years	Can function with understanding. Enjoy things they have always enjoyed - watch TV, play and listen to music, play games.
	Can no longer hold a job, plan and prepare meals, handle personal finances, etc. Driving becomes difficult although can drive to familiar places.	4	8 - 12 years	Can still enjoy simple games, watch TV and videos. Enjoys family photos and memories.

Stage	Alzheimer's Disease-Related Dementias (ADRD)	Stage*	Developmental Age*	Diversion/Distraction Activities
Moderate	Can no longer select proper clothing for occasion or season. Needs help to remain safe in home. Forgets to bathe.	5	5 - 7 years	Needs age appropriate toys and games.
	Requires assistance with dressing.	6a	5 years	Enjoy many of the same activities as preschoolers.
	Requires assistance with bathing.	6b	4 years	
	Can no longer use toilet without assistance.	6c	4 years	
	Urinary incontinence	6d	3 - 4 years	
	Fecal incontinence	6e	2 - 3 years	
Severe	Speech now limited to six or so words per day.	7a	15 months	Enjoys infant toys, mobiles, dangling ribbons.
	Speech now limited to one word per day.	7b	1 year	
	Can no longer walk without assistance.	7c	1 year	
	Can no longer sit up without assistance.	7d	6 - 10 months	
	Can no longer smile.	7e	2 - 4 months	
	Can no longer hold up head.	7f	1 - 3 months	

*Based on Functional Assessment Staging Test (FAST).

Note how seven stages delineate how the body shuts down inexorably until infancy is recognizable and the former adult no longer exists as formerly known.

Carolyn you will see, as I did, as she descended that ladder of seven steps.

First, let me remind you that when Carolyn had that break with reality - not knowing me as her husband of 44 years - I had no idea that she was in Stage 1 of Alzheimer's. Secondly, when we all learned from a PET scan the diagnosis, I for one knew little of what that retrogenesis chart contains.

I knew vaguely about what is described as the first three stages of the chart, and that knowledge came from the popularizations of the TV movie of Glen Campbell and the book and movie of the same name *Still Alice*. In those stories both principal characters have Alzheimer's.

I became acquainted with the chart 20 months after Carolyn was diagnosed with the lethal disease, Alzheimer's. Up to then the degree of uncertainty of what to expect next was considerably higher than after I had this as a road map.

It is my firm intention to place this information here, with the permission of its author, as a heads-up to future unsuspecting caregivers of Alzheimer's patients so that your limbo is less fraught with the major uncertainties especially when the journey begins.

Before the formal diagnosis was rendered, I struggled with what to call what appeared like a break with reality on Carolyn's part. Actually, there existed two breaks for which I searched for answers: what to call her break with reality and the simultaneous break of my heart.

Awareness of these two breaks alerted me to attend to her woundedness and to mine. I credit my past profession for allowing me to know that a caretaker needs to know to take care of him/her self to maintain equilibrium. Without equilibrium, a caretaker is not at his or her best.

I instinctively recoiled from calling Carolyn's lack of recognition for me "a break with reality" because, in my own profession as a psychotherapist for 31 years, a break with reality means: insanity, psychosis, and craziness. Those terms label an extremely harsh reality and not one I wanted to ascribe to Carolyn. I did not want, for an instant, to believe that the woman I had had as a wife for 44 years was insane, crazy, and/or psychotic. I was plain scared.

She did not look insane.

She did not look crazy.

She did not look psychotic.

She looked to me as a perfectly sane Carolyn who simply did not know who I was and that was because what I looked like to her was not what her Edward looked like. "Other than that, there was no psychosis there in front of me," I told myself.

Was I juggling contradictions? Of course, I was juggling contradictions, but I did not for a long while know what else to do. Actually, I determined much later that my contradictory behavior reflected her contradictory "normalcy" in everything except in her abnormalcy in not knowing that I was Edward.

In time, as she began her descent into retrogenesis, Carolyn lost more and more normalcy and exhibited less and less sanity. The downward spiral began approximately one month after the major break of May 12, 2012. In that month, I was reminded of an episode which had had nothing to do with the major break yet turned out to be a harbinger of Capgras. The harbinger or fore-runner of the first Capgras event occurred five months prior in December of 2011.

It was two or three days before Christmas that year, and she and I were driving into Montgomery and Titus, Alabama, to celebrate that holiday with family whom we inherited from her brother's marriage. By then her brother, Ken, whom she adored, had died. But during his lifetime, Carolyn and myself both developed enormously strong ties with her brother's family - wife, Cookie, and daughters, Eileen and Emily, and the spouses and kids of both those dear nieces - as they grew into womanhood and marriage.

The trip to Montgomery entails leaving San Antonio on Highway I-10 and heading towards where the sun rises faithfully every 24 hours to make it daylight in our part of the world. We proceeded east on I-10 to Mobile, Alabama, after stopping once to sleep. Once in Mobile, the direction we sought was a hard left onto highway I-65 towards Montgomery.

From that Mobile juncture, one is on the home stretch to Montgomery, our destination that day in late December. It amounts to approximately 173 miles of easy traveling from Mobile and is usually as pleasant as any road lined on both sides of the highway by pine trees and copious greenery - all a normal, ordinary drive.

We had made the trip close to dozens of times, enough to recognize the landmarks which, of course, are verified by highway signs for which the U.S. interstate highway system is well appreciated.

About one month after we were visited with the upending of our lives by Capgras, I began to recall with great interest the details of that December 2011 trip. As we approached the juncture where we would turn left onto I-65, Carolyn asked quizzically: "Who tells us where to turn?" The question threw me, I asked: "Pardon me?"

She repeated what I thought I had heard but could not comprehend why she was asking: "Who tells us where to turn?" "I mean, when do they tell us?"

I responded as if I were calm (but inside of myself, I was incredulous that I had heard from her what I thought I had just heard with my disbelieving ears): "Well, we know to turn on I-65 when we get to the outskirts of Mobile." Her questioning continued: "How will we know when to turn?" "Won't someone tell us?"

I again tried reassuringly (I truly believed) to tell her that we'd know from the signs where to turn (I chided myself to stop it and not be alarmed by these - at worst - simplistic questions.)

By that time, we had begun seeing the highway signs for the tourist center "up ahead." It was one we had frequented in the past, if for nothing else, to use the bathrooms and exercise our legs before the final stretch which was to begin right ahead at the outskirts of Mobile. She then began asking: "Will they know at the tourist center where we are supposed to turn?" "Will they have maps they can give us?"

She knew that the tourist center specialized in map giving, but it seemed as if she were trying to be gentle with me in case I did not know that they had maps or as if I had forgotten that. As these odd questions continued, I knew something was off and I could not understand why there was mounting anxiety in her voice. One of my treatment specialties had been anxiety and panic attacks. I knew I was hearing anxiety in her questions but it did not seem appropriate for grown woman Carolyn. Had she been a child of maybe eight or nine, her questions and commensurate anxiety would have been very age-appropriate.

Inside of myself I did not want to label what I was witnessing as "mounting anxiety" of the pathological type, i.e. when it is too high, too frequent or too long lasting, much less did I want to betray to her that I had a mounting concern. Ah ha! I was having my own mounting anxiety for I feared, fear. Not only was I afraid, I was fearing my being afraid. So, I gave in without a struggle and said: "Yes, we can go in and ask for directions as to where to turn to go to Montgomery."

That satisfied her immensely! That we were going to ask and be told "where to turn" and "how to go." (She was satisfied as a frightened little child of eight or nine would have been to have her fears alleviated.) Mine were not; without giving it words in my own self I was intuiting that her behavior was that of an eight-year-old. So we stopped, and a very courteous attendant showed us on an enormous map of the territory where I-10 and I-65 intersected and how we would make that turn before going into the city of Mobile so as to avoid city traffic.

We departed the tourist center armed with one more Alabama map as we already had one in the glove compartment. When we approached our intended cut-off from I-10 to head north, she became increasingly (almost jubilant) joyful that: "Uh huh, we were finally coming to it."

I agreed that, indeed, we were closer and then proceeded to get on to I-65; we were barely seeing the rural part of the city of Mobile on our right-hand side as we headed north.

Very quickly she blurted out, "Here, we have to turn here (pointing to the east). We are here; we have to turn on one of these roads that you are passing. Here's where we go to Cookie's house."

She kept repeating this message with more and more alarm in her voice because I kept heading north. I was denying everything she was saying by replying: "No, we aren't there yet. That is the rural outskirt of Mobile." At first I was impatient at her insistence but still using a calm voice. My calm voice was not working. Because I was not turning, she perceived that our chance for getting to Cookie's was being lost. She told me in no uncertain terms how she and her brother knew this territory better than I did. She knew where we were supposed to turn.

She was lost "as to place" yet believed that I was the one who was lost and told me so with more and more anger because she believed I was ignoring her commands to turn east. Once her nervousness turned to anxiousness and her anxiety became panic, she fell into anger and commanded me to "stop the car."

I kept insisting as I kept driving, "Honey, we are still 173 miles from Montgomery; this is Mobile we are passing." "Carolyn, I am not lost."

I began pointing to the highway signs which said Montgomery 173 miles... 170 miles... 165... etc.

She then began to accuse me in angry tones of going in "circles" because she could recognize that we had already passed through our surroundings earlier. Then she went on to say, "I don't care what the signs say; my brother and I know this part of the country." She again commanded and begged that I stop the car, saying that she needed to get out because I was bypassing where we were supposed to be going. As soon as I heard her say: "I don't care what the signs say," I realized this was craziness talking and it petrified me. I instinctively did not want to stop the car because I knew from her erratic behavior that I would not have the ability to persuade her to come back in unless I used physical force.

Physical force was the last thing I wanted to try on her. We were still in a somewhat populated area, and, to onlookers, me forcing her into the car would appear like physical abuse in action.

She was experiencing "disorientation as to place," and I knew it but she did not. She did not know she was lost, and that bit of reality was a huge mountain of worry to my denying self. I could not believe what I was witnessing. It was one of those experiences which you know can happen, but you never believed it would happen to you nor to your spouse of 40 some years.

People casually label these type of moments insane moments. This was truly being experienced by me as an insane moment and I still had over 160 miles of trying to contain the moment or diffuse the moment. I had already given up trying to understand the moment.

I knew three things for certain: keep driving, do not stop this car for anything, and insist on the rationality of the highway signs even if she cannot - and who knows why. Much later I realized I had been coaching myself to stay sane.

Her degree of confusion confused me enormously. I could not understand why she dismissed the "objective reality" of highway signs that said, "Montgomery: 170 miles or 167 miles, etc.'"

In my total astonishment about her behavior, I did not avert to the fact that I was feeding fear on top of fear by taking her further and further from the place where she was iron-clad convinced we needed to be. All I saw was anger on top of anger. Irrational on top of irrational.

I had been full of fear once upon a time, back in 1967 (44 years prior to all of this) when I was experiencing panic attacks of the crippling kind; on second thought, all panic attacks are, indeed, crippling because in their presence one is incapable of normal functioning.

My moments of panic back then seemed like eternal moments. They were so unknown to me (as they are to all first-time sufferers) and were so severe that I immediately believed that I was literally losing my mind. I felt "insanity!" "This is what insanity feels like," I had pronounced to myself.

A prime symptom which I experienced - but not all panic attackers experience it - goes by the euphemism "light-headed." Technically, psychology brands this symptom as derealization or depersonalization. It manifests itself as if the mind is leaving one's body. It can feel like the part of one who is conscious (the mind) is either going sideways out of the head and body or (more commonly for me) that the mind is traveling ever so slowly, but incrementally and assuredly out from the top of the skull to who-knows-where-it-is-going! It is to experience the most frightening thing: that one has absolutely no control over any of what is transpiring and nothing about it is positive in any imaginable way.

Actually, in 1967, I experienced panic attacks four distinct times and each time I believed I was going crazy. When the attack was over or when my mind "magically" returned to its place within me, I believed I had returned to sanity.

Though the events of 1967 were, as of this writing, 50 years ago, I can still remember the vividness of that experience when I was 33 years old.

Upon reflection of this December 2011 event of Carolyn's, as I was recalling it a month or so after Capgras, I began to arrive upon the realization that she must have been going through the same trauma as I had gone through when I was in fear of fear. When she was in that state, what I picked up was her anger.

At the time, what I experienced quite profoundly in the December 2011 event was the bruising and woundedness of my ego at the mercy of her domineering anger.

More bizarre happenings were to come in that trek between Mobile and our final destination which followed a trajectory totally unsatisfactory to both of us in two separate realities. Carolyn had a sudden keen interest in the I-65 bridge that crosses the Tensaw River delta north of Mobile.

She had continued to chide, scold, and mimic me for "going in circles" (which accounted for why we weren't there yet) and then interrupted this line of beratement with: "Where's the bridge?" "Why haven't we passed the bridge?" "Did we pass the bridge?"

After gathering my bearings, I answered, "Yes, I remember a bridge, it must be up ahead because, no, we haven't passed the bridge yet." Again, her sarcastic explanation was that if I would stop going in circles, I would have gotten to it. It would be in the following months that she would nonchalantly tell me that her interest in the bridge at that time had been because she anticipated jumping off it! Never did that occur to me when we were going through that jungle of strangeness that Carolyn was irrational enough to want to end it all with a jump off a bridge easily 40 stories high.

What occasioned the nonchalant revelation, besides the obvious elusiveness of the danger portended by that event for her, was that for a series of reasons we had come to believe that that whole December 2011 bizarreness was triggered by her receiving a medication for a hypothyroid condition which was the wrong and potentially lethal dose for her. In that context of how bizarre and frightening that all was when we "chatted about it" months later, she casually let me know "how" she had experienced the lethality of a wrong medication. She told me of wanting to end that event by jumping off the I-65 bridge.

And to think! I was so glad when we got to that bridge because, then, I thought of it as "something amidst all this turmoil to make her happy." No, she never attempted to jump. The 65 or 70 MPH of our Nissan Maxima going across that bridge precluded any such thought; little did I know.

She managed to outlive her panic state and anger state as awareness sunk in that we were indeed side-stepping Montgomery and were within a stone's throw of our destination, Cookie's lakeside home in Titus where the Christmas crowd awaited our arrival after two or three phone contacts to correct our course through that beautiful rural countryside (which kinda, sort of resembled the outskirts of rural Mobile, but not really).

Once we arrived she just accepted that we were there. No recriminations, no apologies, no search for answers for all that emotional upheaval. She did none of this; neither did I.

I was ever grateful to the Conscious Universe (of the Creator, of course) that we had arrived and that, strangely enough, we were out of strangeness. I did not want to awaken a panic or anger which suddenly went dormant.

So, I said nothing of that daytime nightmare.

We both tried to muster up our usual non-harried demeanor, and it worked. No one suspected what I later repeated to them. They were aghast and equally appalled that "the wrong meds" can wreak chaos.

The detail which I have chosen to give to this harbinger of Capgras is to demonstrate again that it is painfully erroneous to believe that an Alzheimer's patient does not suffer as much as the caregiver does. In the first stages of retrogenesis Carolyn suffered immeasurably, and I, with all my training and experience of 31 years as a psychotherapist, was in for one rollercoaster ride after another. On a rollercoaster you know there's a drop at the peak of the ascent, but your adrenaline mechanism is never quite prepared enough to completely arrest "fight or flight" when one knows not what to fight for nor what to flee from. That alone compounds the attack stage; it evokes more adrenaline in the system. And adrenaline always works; it always heightens heart rate. The heart rate increases blood flow and accompanying oxygen to all cells for more energy with which to meet whatever is being perceived as danger to the organism, and the mind is yelling (not whispering) "fight or flee." But as I say, when one does not know what the enemy is to be fought nor what one is to flee from, that alone is perceived as real danger, triggering off more adrenaline and a vicious cycle becomes one of panic or anxiety attack stage wherein one feels paralyzed. Some feel like jumping off a 40-story bridge!!

CHAPTER FOUR
THE REVELATION OF THE MOMENT

Obviously, it is one thing to know all of any of this clinically; it is quite another to be experiencing it over and over again. This is exactly what we were in for during the 19 months following the first signs of Capgras from May 12, 2012, to February 13, 2014. As abnormally as this whole episode evolved, I had no inkling it signaled the beginning of a lethal disease.

In the first two to three months after Capgras set in, Carolyn knew "who I was" about as many days as she took me to be a stranger who would appear when her husband disappeared. She might know me as Edward for three days and then be asking: "Where did Edward go?" Every time she would recognize me again, the event brought joy at seeing me and recrimination for having gone away and not letting her know I was going to go. She delighted in my return but could not stop herself from chiding me for having left her to fend for herself with those strangers who claimed to also be called Ed or Edward.

For me too there was joy at being recognized for who I was but there was pain too; pain for having to explain where or why I had gone when, obviously, I had gone nowhere. This reality she was increasingly less able to comprehend.

The duration of time between Capgras episodes could be one or two days or three or four weeks. The Capgras episode itself, too, could last two or three days before she'd "see" me as the Edward she had married.

The quality of those episodes varied too. At times Carolyn treated me as if I were someone older than the husband who disappeared. Often that stranger appeared younger or older than he had the last time she perceived that stranger to have been with her.

"Where is your father?" she would ask me, as I were a perfect stranger to her and the person she was inquiring about was one with whom she had interacted recently. That's how I came to realize that her question was not about my real father whom she met many years ago before he had died.

Likewise, she frequently asked, "Where is your son? I was just talking to him...?" At times, she reported that she had just communicated with the other Ed that morning only yesterday, and, since we did not have a son, I knew it was not a living person from our life whom she had dealt with.

It took me some time to figure out that when Carolyn "saw" a stranger that stranger took multiple forms; for her there were times when the stranger had been a woman.

"Where is that woman who was talking to me about my meds at the kitchen table?" She would ask this when it had been she and I talking about these meds at our kitchen table. Or she would ask, "That woman who was just here; where did she go?" and it had been me with her. On several occasions, which were scary ones, Carolyn could have sworn that a strange woman had been in bed with me. As she passed by the guest bedroom where I had slept one night, she saw a woman next to me in bed with her arm draped over my body. Another time, when she had gotten up to take her meds at 5:00 a.m. and I had not, she came back to the bed where we had been sleeping together and asked: "Where'd the woman go."

What made those two incidents so scary, was the anger evoked in her when I went on to quietly tell her there had been no other woman with me in bed. She was furious with me for my denial and her expressed anger scared me because I was feeling anger directed at me as if I were a lying, cheating S.O.B.

The advice: "Don't take it personally" does absolutely no good under the circumstances. Of course, she was not to blame for her behavior. I could not blame her, but neither could I not feel what was personally directed at me.

At the beginning months of Capgras's comings and goings, Carolyn challenged me about calling myself Edward. She came around to just being amazed and amazed that there existed so many Edwards. The fact that she saw so many Edwards betrayed that she saw more than one stranger in place of Edward - her husband - but never more than one at a time.

If you have taken time to imagine your loved one of many years asking you, on a perfectly normal, average, common, garden-variety evening, "What is your name?" and "Who are you?" and, if you can give yourself license to imagine how the rest of the moments in your life are transformed - totally transformed - by an episode of that ilk, try imagining the scariness you might experience - regardless of your gender - when that loved one takes to awakening you from sound sleep in the middle of the night or before the cocks crow the arrival of dawn to ask: "What is your name?" "How did you get here?" "Who are you?"

In this scenario (which happened more times than I care to remember) when Capgras intruded Carolyn's space irrespective of time of day or night, it was scary for a number of reasons. For one, I never knew, when so awakened, how long she might have been staring at me in the dark with flashlight in hand puzzling as to who I might be. Nor did I know how scared or threatened she was feeling at say 2:00 a.m. or 4:30 a.m. Once we turned on the light to converse and address her question, I had no idea how amenable she would be to my responses which never carried the solution she so desperately wanted. There was never a solution to her quandary.

There was always the possibility for violence, although past experiences kept reminding me the probability was low, but at 2:00 or 4:30 a.m. I never knew.

Also, the degree of her wakefulness (her wake-full state) would determine how long into the night or early morning we would have to negotiate that given experience. I could not help but wonder whether the companion queries would arise, like: "Where then is Edward?" "Do you know here he is?" "Is this a game you are playing?" "Well, who sent you and why?"

If she did have these questions also disturbing her existence, it was imperative that I be up for as long as it took to bring some semblance of contentedness to her mind so that she might be able to return to needed nighttime sleep. It goes without saying, that I, too, needed that nighttime sleep.

Some of the times, the tone of her voice and in her voice led me to gauge the degree of fear she might be experiencing (like on a "1" to "10" scale with "10" being the highest, any fear above a "7" is incapacitating; a fear from "4" to "6" is beginning to be alarming and is beginning to interfere with judgement making. A fear from "1" to "3" is normal i.e., not pathological.) I knew from my past professional practice as a behavior and cognitive modification specialist that fear (anxiety) comes in the three parameters of frequency, intensity, and duration.

The better I could help her arrest the intensity (before it reached pathologic proportions) the lower the duration of fear for that episode and also the less disturbing memories of that episode would be thus cutting into the frequency. Every episode was unique unto itself, meaning that there existed a history of her being unable to develop the skill of arresting the intensity of her fears based on her past experiences. She was not retaining the memory of those episodes. I felt I had to guide her to bring down the fear every time she began to exhibit it. At 2:00 a.m. or 4:30 a.m., this was always considerately more of a challenge. Wonderful to report that she never did get violent and, truthfully, I can say she was cooperative in arresting that intensity before it climbed to panic or anxiety attack state many a time. That made life a bit more bearable both for her and for me or other caregivers.

That this became exhausting is an understatement - the challenge for the caregiving person to be on alert for the presence of fear in her perception of her new reality.

In the early stages of Capgras and the awakening in the middle of the night, I would have been foolish to not wonder whether it was safe for me to go to sleep there in that home (our home). "Could she do something lethal to me while I slept?" Of course, it was possible. I never had reason to believe that she probably would harm me.

When friends and relatives asked, "Are you safe there?" I knew they, too, could not dismiss the possible. Thankfully, I was never threatened. She learned to trust me. My many prayers were answered in so many ways amidst the chaos - the indisputable chaos - in our lives.

A few months into the Capgras syndrome, she would ask, "Where are the others?" Often this occurred when we were about to sit down to eat. I would respond at the beginning of this series of occurrences, "What others?" and she was never able to give names of who she thought should be there to eat with us, if she answered anything, because frequently all she did was give me a blank stare. As if I should know who the others were, she would exclaim: "The others!"

Later, I learned to handle this question about others with: "It is just you and me, Carolyn." Some of the times she would simply dismiss the incident with that reply, at other times she would walk past me and go poke her head in the TV room or the living room. Having found no one, she would just sit down with me to eat; it was up to me to begin the next conversation, if there were to be any at that meal time.

On occasion, she pointed to the hallway closet door thinking there was a staircase behind it which led to a basement, as if that was where "the others" were. We had no basement. Only one of the 10 homes we ever lived in had a basement and that antedated this period of time by more than 30 years.

There were times when the confusion of people living downstairs caused her to scold me for not keeping their racket under control. She said more than once, "You say you are here to help me and you don't listen to me say, 'They are making noise and you do not stop them.'" I would ask, "When did you hear the noise?" My questions were always answered with the same quizzical look she'd give me when I asked: "What others?"

In time I learned to realize that, more and more frequently, she was forgetting what she had just said just as quickly as it took her to ask a question. Her quizzicalness was there, apparently, because she literally had no idea of the context of my question which was of course the question she had posed in the first place. It was as if I had posed an abstract question from out of nowhere.

The realizations that came with repetitive incidents like these did not make each incident any less strange when it again happened. The subject of "others" was always a strange phenomenon to work through with her in such a way as to not make her feel like she was "crazy" or "not normal."

I wanted her to feel ever so normal and loved. I never believed I could "love her back to normalcy" but I did hope with intensity that something would spring normalcy back into her life just like "something" frequently brought her out of Capgras and she knew me as her husband - even if it were "just" for a while.

At times, when Capgras had been going on for a prolonged period of time - say two to three weeks without interruption - she would treat the circumstance of us in the same house without the presence of her husband as a curious evolvement that she must have consented to but had no recollection of it. In a friendly manner she would ask, "Did they send you here to, as you say, take care of me?"

A variation to that question was: "Who was it to ask you to come here?" (sic) There would be no anger nor recrimination in her tone of voice. It was as if she should know but just didn't. At times she would ask: "So who is it you work for?" Or she would be talking of the "several of us who came and went" and inquire: "What type of company is it that you all work for?"

At these times, I found myself walking a tight rope of not wanting to feed more fuel to her delusion, i.e., not wanting to suggest that we were in separate realities. I would say, "I am here because I choose to be here to help you" or "...because I want to make sure you are ok going to see doctor so and so..." or "...because I know you want help with all those medicines you have to take so early, and I know how confusing it can all get." I picked on something that both of our realities agreed upon, as it were.

A strange sensation occurred inside of me every time she would tell me of a conversation she had had with me but she believed she was dealing with two separate persons. What she recounted in these instances was always faithful to how I had experienced it (the last time!) and it revealed to me an impression she had experienced which I would have never known about.

I am trying to convey that, no matter how many times I experienced being treated by my own spouse as if I were a total stranger, it felt very surreal to realize: she truly does not see the "me" standing right here. I never felt: this is normal. The awareness of that was just that, an awareness; it was not terrifying anymore, it was not a subject for tears, nor hair pulling after a while. It was "just" an awareness of something of awe. Again, I knew it was possible for this to happen to us but I never believed it would, so, every time it happened it acutely awoke me to being awake.

By now, it should be evident that there was nothing simple about dealing with Carolyn's experience of Capgras. It was not a simple "she got to where she did not 'see' her husband Edward when she saw me." You, the reader can now see how many things Capgras entailed. She never could capture the meaning of Capgras even though it appeared for a long time when all else was normal, that is, when she could be rational about so much in life. Her psychiatrist explained Capgras to her in simple terms with me present. She was given written information about how it constituted a delusion due to cognitive dysfunction and not a hallucination.

The little Carolyn managed to grasp was that I, Edward the stranger, brought Capgras into her life. She was pretty sure I could not help doing it but I was the one responsible for it. By the time she came up with this misconception, I had learned that rational explanations went nowhere with the degree of cognitive dysfunction she was experiencing, so I never discussed with her any more than what the psychiatrist had tried to instill in her comprehension. There were times when she wanted me to explain why I had done this to her i.e., brought Capgras which had caused so much pain.

CHAPTER FIVE
THE BACKGROUND OF THE MOMENT

In the meantime, I depended on Carolyn's primary doctor to help me navigate these strange events which wove in and out of sanity and its opposite, but which I was unconsciously resisting to label as insane.

Deep inside of me was the commonplace knowledge that in both the family of her mother and the family of her dad there were sad cases of Alzheimer's. On her mom's side there had been an aunt whom Carolyn loved dearly and on her dad's side his only brother had been stricken by the disease. Carolyn had suffered seeing that uncle was so far into retrogenesis at the time of Carolyn's dad's death that he was not aware he was at a funeral - the funeral of his only brother.

In my general knowledge of Alzheimer's I knew it was hereditary and, Carolyn, who had done extensive work with geriatric populations (as a Director of Admissions at a place that featured custodial care in Independent Living, Assisted Living, and a nursing home including an Alzheimer's unit) also knew it was hereditary, but we never said out loud that we feared it might visit her. It had not visited her brother who was older and had died of cancer.

Not talking about it, obviously, did not make the possibility nor the probability nor the certainty less real, but I had considered the possibility. I deliberately did not discuss the possibility to prevent the anticipatory anxiety which I believed it would bring. To this day, I do not regret that decision.

Her primary had already been dealing with Carolyn's symptoms of cognitive dysfunction and had managed to convince Carolyn that to admit to that diagnosis, cognitive dysfunction, was not tantamount to admitting anything other than that she was having the problems many seniors begin to experience when they forget words. Carolyn learned to call it "dropping words." She was comfortable calling it that but it caused her much anxiety that nothing was dispelling the word dropping.

She began to think that the dysfunction was due to her having resigned her position as Director of Admissions at Morningside Manor. She also developed the belief that I was the one who insisted on her resigning that position. I heard her tell many a person to whom she confessed her total regret that she had retired that I wanted her retired so that we could take trips abroad.

I hated to contradict her because the painful reality which I had witnessed, in her last two years on the job, was that the work she loved had started to become a tremendous source of anxiety and anger. She was coming home every evening uptight with bodily stress and mental anxiety. As she related each evening what was evoking these emotions she became increasingly more and more angry.

She resented the direction towards which the agency was heading, as more programs had to be sacrificed to money matters. For instance, the number of Medicaid beds began to be curtailed because the cost of living was putting pressure on the organization to meet budget. The Medicaid reimbursement to her institution was too low so those beds were turned to bigger money makers. This rancored her soul when she saw poorer people unable to afford her agency's services.

Her anger found an easy target in the administrators who changed agency policy. To Carolyn's way of thinking, these administrators did this at the expense of the agency's mission.

For her to experience the mission being changed was tantamount to betrayal of fundamental values. This anger never let up.

There was, too, more emphasis on the use of computers in Carolyn's work. Everyone's job descriptions at Morningside Manor were being re-written to reflect this needed skill. This affected her directly and meant that she was expected to spend more time recording in computer files and less time on one-to-one encounters. She had for years prided herself on the personal touch that can happen with one-to-one contact. Now, the clear signal was "put data into the computer and the necessary segments of the organization can read it for themselves." Along with this there were demands put on her office to be at the "beck and call" of the marketing department which, in her eyes, took her office away from service to people.

For reasons like these I did encourage her to retire once she completed her tenth year in that position; the position was changing because all of life was changing at the lightning speed which the computer brought into being.

She continued believing that, had she not retired, she would not have begun the memory problems which word dropping indicated. So, to her, word dropping was Edward's fault. That, of course, hurt both of our egos tremendously.

It goes without saying that the more pronounced cognitive dysfunction became the less she was to blame for what or how she perceived.

I began the process of writing hand-written, four to five page letters to her primary and then hand delivering them one day prior to each of Carolyn's appointments. The letters were a progress report on everything from the frequency of Capgras to the fidelity of taking medications and, in general, the degree of cognitive dysfunction from visit to visit.

Fortunately, Carolyn allowed me to go into her visits with her primary and, subsequently, with her psychiatrist and then also to her neurologist whom the primary had succeeded in getting Carolyn to agree to start seeing on a regular basis for help with the word dropping.

In my professional life I had dealt with those two professionals - the psychiatrist whom Carolyn saw weekly and the neurologist whom she saw perhaps once a month for follow up evaluations - and I knew their reputations in their respective fields to excel among their peers.

It gratified me tremendously that Carolyn was in the hands of excellent and competent professionals. Although it totally surprised me that the twists and turns of the disease Alzheimer's were so unpredictable, even to them, that none of her doctors could give guidance as to when was it indicated that she would require in-patient treatment and if so what type. Nursing home? Or assisted living? Or other? What other was there? The doctors were in limbo but I felt my limbo was more acute since I was her primary caregiver and more and increasingly more in charge of her daily life. Her psychiatrist and neurologist, too, would receive from me a progress report, in the frankest of terms so that they had a clearer idea of her progress or lack thereof than had they had to depend on her inability to self-report.

As the obituary at the front end of this saga indicated, Carolyn's parents and grandparents, as well as aunts and uncles on both sides of her family all preceded her in death, so her remaining family consisted of two sisters from her mom's second marriage, a brother-in-law married to one of those sisters, four nieces, and her sister-in-law Cookie. There was, too, one cousin whom Carolyn regarded more like an aunt due to her seniority and the relationship that Carolyn had had with that cousin's mother. There were distant cousins in other cities.

Of the few relatives who remained to witness her path through retrogenesis, only one lived in our city of residence, San Antonio. That was Carolyn's youngest sister, Lisa, whom she had helped raise and whom Carolyn adored.

There existed a number of women who remained in touch over the years as dear friends in the city. Another group existed in places where we had lived formerly and with whom the ties of friendship never eroded.

In the time frame from May 12, 2012, to July of that year we had no diagnosis until the results came in from one PET scan ordered by her primary physician.

Unfortunately, her primary was not in town for the office visit which was scheduled for discussion of what the PET scan revealed.

What rendered it unfortunate and akin to a disaster was that the nurse practitioner, whom Carolyn had never seen and had had no opportunity to develop confidence in, was the one to unceremoniously blurted out to my wife: "You have a brain pattern consistent with Alzheimer's." Carolyn, with incredulity, blurted back "What?" And the nurse practitioner defensively shot the hurtful phrase back: "You have Alzheimer's."

I hurt for my wife and for me in that acrimonious exchange of two seconds which presaged the pains of retrogenesis for Sara Carolyn Alderette (those two seconds defined much of the next three to four months.) Carolyn's recovery from that last volley of shot gun blast at point-blank range took the form of something like: "You know nothing about me. I will wait to discuss this with (my primary) when she returns." With that, Carolyn bolted out and left. The nurse practitioner gave me the written PET scan report which Carolyn refused to take from her extended hand.

Carolyn's denial was swift and strong enough to never, ever retract it. I never pressed her to do so either. She never pronounced: "I do not have Alzheimer's." Neither did she ever ask: "Do I have it?" Nor did she ask: "What do I have?" I knew immediately and said to myself, "I cannot deny this reality. I now focus on taking care of her more and more because Alzheimer's is a progressive disease." I wrote to her doctors whom I informed of the disastrous turn of events with that one nurse practitioner.

In their early assessment, neither the psychiatrist nor the neurologist found evidence of Alzheimer's underneath the detected cognitive dysfunction. In those early stages, they were not calling Capgras by that name. They had no idea what to account for the phenomenon. From the beginning, it was not straight-up not recognizing Edward. It was a serious phenomenon.

In the meantime, instinct alone told me to keep doing the things Edward would do and this with the hope that Carolyn would see familiar acts in a familiar environment that would/could trigger whatever the perception mechanism her brain needed to perceive that it was indeed Edward she saw carrying on. The only consistency I saw in the pattern was that when Capgras ceased, I appeared to her perception: when "it" or Capgras happened, I disappeared (obviously). But to Carolyn this realization of pattern could not occur. She never "saw" that stranger(s) and Edward never appeared together. Many times when I returned to her perception as me she would tell me about when she had believed I was someone other than myself.

Some people whom I could talk to about what was going on had the naiveté to ask, "Are you sure she is not putting you on?" They actually believed she engaged in the same cruelty which she, at times, accused me of. The point is that, sometimes, well-intentioned friends and/or relatives cause more pain than healing with their naiveté.

More pain and fear appeared on her calendar every time Capgras appeared anew because each such return was fraught with the same questions: "Where is Edward?" "Does he not love me?" "Is that why he left?" or "What did you do to him?" "Is he alive?" "Do you know where he is?" etc. I began to notice that she started not knowing that she had had this experience of Edward's disappearance. Each time it began to feel like the first time to her.

This angle of the phenomenon of Capgras manifested itself in occasions such as the time when I first noticed that she could not tie her shoe laces (anymore). Thing was she had no realization that she had known how to tie shoe laces at one time. She experienced that inability as if she had never known how to. She was in that instance like a child of five or six. On one occasion she expressed wonder and admiration that I knew how to make up a bed. There, too, she lacked the awareness that she had had that ability. She assumed she had not yet learned how to do that.

The point I wish to highlight is that Capgras didn't make her forget certain abilities; it simply erased the skill and any memory of her as the adult who had had those particular skills.

Gradually, she read books less and less, to the point where she read her last book or cooked her last meal or drove her car for the last time or even knew that it was she who brought her car to her garage when in total amazement she asked me (for the first time) "Who brought my car to this garage?" She had no idea she had driven it there.

These were painful-to-the-gut moments for me when I experienced her for the first time doing something for the last time.

It was only later of course that I could look back and note when it was that she had done such and such for the very last time. Simple things were no longer simple. They were things of the past. They no longer existed.

Every one of those moments called for the compassionate response on all our parts, from me especially since I was with her 24/7 for the first 19 months after Capgras appeared. We needed to treat her at the state she was in and in no way suggest that she needed to know how to do or want to know how to do such and such. We guided her through the episode which she was experiencing as "mysterious" in a manner much like one does with five or six-year-olds when facing a thing not understood.

Carolyn herself had demonstrated precisely that compassionate response to many an Alzheimer's patient at her place of employment in the Alzheimer's unit at Morningside Manor. She had always known how to make the helpless feel hopeful in one way or another, just like she had instinctively known how to bring strength to the geriatric people she loved and who were demonstrating weakness or scared feelings brought on by confusion over not knowing or comprehending events current in their lives.

This marked contrast wasn't lost on people close to her who had witnessed the nurturance and affection she had displayed towards senior citizens in Dementia. They were now experiencing her, Carolyn, in Dementia (of the Alzheimer's type). Their hurt was there in the open.

In the early stages of cognitive dysfunction, Carolyn was aware enough to know how those early malfunctions could be omens of the harsh condition she had helped Alzheimer's patients deal with. She said nothing out loud of her fear; what betrayed the presence of that fear was her growing anxiety related to the frequency, intensity, and duration of these malfunctions. The higher it was in all three of these parameters, the more the dysfunction manifested itself. The flip-side of this coin was that the deeper she went into retrogenesis the less aware she was of what was transforming her and this resulted in less anxiety manifesting itself. This was a strange but true-to-life paradox.

She and I and her mom and two sisters had seen this type of progression in Carolyn's step father when he first developed Dementia. When first placed in an Alzheimer's unit, he made his displeasure well known for the visitors terminating their visits. As the disease took a firmer hold, the less aware he was of what might trigger fear and he consequently experienced nothing of the sort in the latter stages of retrogenesis.

In that whole journey of her stepfather, Carolyn had shown tremendous affection and compassion not only for him but for her mom, as well, who needed assistance to better take care of herself for her own sake and for the sake of being a responsible and able caregiver.

I mention this and her history of working in the care of patients in Dementia to point out that in the early stages of her disease when she still had the awareness of how dreadful it can all be and when in all likelihood she did dread it for herself, none of her previous contacts with the process gave her any clue of how to accept it gracefully or without fear. But let me repeat, the fear did lessen as she proceeded the path down Alzheimer's road - an inexorable procession.

I would be remiss if I failed to acknowledge and to thank the numerous friends and family who sincerely told us of their many prayers for Carolyn and for me. Those reminders served as exhortations for me to ask for strength, courage, humility, and patience. They enabled me to absorb the berating and the accusations and to stay quiet, calm, and present in knowing full well that defensiveness was the last thing I needed to engage in. I needed the Divine in order to be able to be on her side, even when she was seeing me as the cause of her misery.

CHAPTER SIX
THE REALITY OF THE MOMENT

By the third or fourth month after Capgras appeared - approximately August or September of 2012 - I realized that every indication of her "being out of our reality" was not an indication that her state of being was a mystery to her. Our reality was a mystery to her - the one she was experiencing, the one she was in, was not mysterious to her any more than the surreal reality which we are in when we are in a dream is to us. We experience what we dream as if it is really happening. The dreamer who is asleep does not know it is a dream he/she is experiencing. The land of the surreal is as real to that dreamer as our reality - in our waking state - is to us.

I say this in as many ways as I do because I discovered that it was highly and critically important for me to acknowledge the reality which was gripping her attention as powerfully as my reality was gripping me, even if she could not communicate to us in our world what the existence was that she was experiencing. This acknowledgement needed to be genuine and in no way condescending any more than we needed to be condescending with the imaginings of a child as we help that child navigate through what is being perceived to have existence in the objective realm.

In the first phase of retrogenesis (the 19 months between May 12, 2012, and February 14, 2014) there were many occasions when I took her to see one of her three doctors: her primary, her psychiatrist, and her neurologist. There were times when she believed that the person accompanying her was me, her husband, and at other times she believed it was someone else. More and more she regarded the someone else as someone she had (fortunately for me) learned to rely on and to do so with trust.

One of these times, to my mild surprise, she answered her primary's question about who was accompanying her with the reply that I was her husband, Edward. "Edward, my husband," she responded without a hesitancy. Upon leaving the doctor's office she confided in me that sometimes she introduced me as her husband because if she were to identify me as someone other, they would think she was crazy (sic).

I managed to hide my amazement that, even in the throes of Capgras, she still had some self-defense mechanisms. This type of episode indicated forcefully how for periods of time in this first phase, she began to be quite comfortable with me being someone other than the "real" Edward.

Nevertheless, she was always delighted with joy and genuine gladness when the real one reappeared.

Her ability to return to recognizing me for who I have always been always happened for random reasons unknown to me much less to her. This perdured from the beginning of retrogenesis to the final end.

More than once she had begun to comment on the coincidence of "so many Edwards." At times, she wondered out loud whether "maybe some of them are liars." And if they were lying, she wondered with great innocence, "Why would they lie?" When she was so puzzled and asked questions like this, expecting me to solve the riddle, I had no ready answer and had to rely on the instinct of the moment for how to respond. Nothing in all of my four careers gave me a clue on how to respond without being disingenuous. I did not want to feed into the delusion as if I believed it to be true, nor did I want to relay any modicum of derision about her delusion which always always was such a real experience of what was, in fact, real to her.

Instinct took me to learn "being quiet" many a time or to say, "I just don't know either." At times I would go for reassurance like: "Carolyn, someday maybe we'll know." Little by little, I, too, became calm in the face of not having answers by cultivating "it's OK not to know." I was able to be less concerned with my ego knowing or not knowing how to negotiate the surprising twists and baffling turns of this journey. The deeper we penetrated this forest the more mysterious it seemed.

When Capgras was a newcomer into both our lives and it would come and go as mentioned earlier, it sometimes took Carolyn a while to forgive me for having gone away or disappeared from one moment (in the kitchen) to the next (in the living room).

At other times, she responded to "his" absence quite calmly, like the times she simply said to my insistence that I was Edward, her husband. "How come I've never seen you before? You must be like a brother my husband had - a brother I never knew about!" She also asked that I not play games with her nor take advantage of her by telling her I was Edward her husband. She stayed on that theme of not knowing me but knowing full well that I could not be her husband Edward. It was as if she were conceding, "OK, you may be Edward, but you are not THE Edward." In that same dialogue and in that same quiet mood she wanted to simply know, "Did he die?" She asked this not with fear or sadness in her voice, only with curiosity. When I perceived this, I felt a tremendous sadness that the prospect of my death was merely a subject of curiosity to my wife. She was of course relating to me, her husband, but she was not knowing it was me; she was demonstrating this curious thing of the possible death of her husband.

My spontaneous physical reaction, before I could take control of my response, was the start of tears in my eyes - not gushing, but undeniably wet tears rolling down my cheek - before I wiped them out of existence.

She had already seen the two or three tears rolling down with tremendous pain and went on to ask: "Why are you crying?" There was human compassion in her voice. She went on to say very sadly: "That isn't fair!" My paraphrase of the rest of her dialogue is that what was unfair was that here she was confronted by the possible death of her husband and deserving of compassion and instead she needed to give compassion to the one taking her husband's place because "he's got tears in his eyes."

With that I felt hotter tears welling up behind and around my eyes. I cannot articulate the pain I experienced with this event any better than through this clumsy analogy of hot tears flowing down with tremendous pain.

Soon after this episode I discontinued arguing my point that, indeed, I was the real Edward. Probably the last time I tried the rational approach to this problem was when I told her that, in the future, recognition of who I was would come to her.

Her unassuming response was: "Are you having a mental problem?" She knew categorically that she was not. And she told me so.

Since I kept insisting on calling myself Ed or Edward - even if not attaching the "I am your husband" part - she wanted to know why I would play such cruelty on her if that was what I was doing. That was one of the many instances she demonstrated that, no, she was not in the reality I was participating in, but I was not in her real reality either. We were in two separate planes of existence; each unable to comprehend the other and each learning, in baby steps, how to accept even that which we did not understand. Just as I was adapting, so was she. (This was a marvelous revelation in the face of the unknowable waterfalls we were headed towards as we proceeded on this river).

Signs of her inner struggles came to me by way of notes I found that she was writing to herself. One such note read and looked like this:

...thoughtful but very hurt by reopening the pain of being an unknown person please don't talk to me re: painful days.

Here is another quote from a notebook that Carolyn used to sometimes journal in. This note of hers shows how a highly educated and articulate woman (who had earned a Masters in Social Work and who had demonstrated a high degree of competency in the various positions alluded to in her obituary) was now losing her ability to communicate with correct grammar.

November 24, 2012

Lisa, Carolyn, and Ed having fun at Esperanza (missed 1st day)
About 6 pm Ed took me to dinner at Luby's
I went to bed, him to T.V.- when I woke up thought he was in bed with me
25th morning became
clear husband had
gone somewhere else
and a person who
claims he is my
husband - who will not come -
this is an issue and
pain a man who is
my husband leaves
house doesn't come
back instead goes
somewhere else

I am close to giving
out.

Although there is no punctuation and subjects and predicates are missing here and there, one can catch the drift of her meaning. But the deficits are glaring.

To be witnessing this befall my wife of 44 years required all the spiritual strength which family and friends promised they were sending. My response to them was to ask them to keep sending what they were promising because somehow it was helping us to stay in this retrogenesis path and find ways and means to serve to the best of our abilities. I say "our" because by now many relatives and friends were very much in evidence and doing what they could when they could. Carolyn and I were never much out of the loving sight of many.

As time passed she was, on the surface, just pleased that I had returned, and there occurred fewer words of recrimination. Under the surface was the reality that she experienced my "absence" with less of a sting and the impostor as more of a matter of fact of her reality. That was the time in this journey when very politely and gently she would ask one of the Edwards: "Who sent you here?" or "What company do you work for?" or "Were you sent to take care of me?" or "Where do you live?" or "Where did you get the keys to the house?" or "Won't they arrest you if you cash a check with Edward's name?"

It almost feels superfluous to say that every day was different. I was always on guard for a new twist in how I needed to relate to her. For example, there were times when it was perfectly "OK" to sleep in the same queen-sized bed as she did but I was always extremely cautious to let her know that I knew to stay at my far end of the bed and knew to never even attempt touching. Over time I gathered that, apparently, she felt safer with someone close by when she fell asleep. She didn't know how to say it but it seemed she wanted protection. (How normal was that!)

At times when her delusions took a different form, she imagined that a woman had been sleeping between us. I know because she would point to the center between us as we awoke and she would quietly ask, "Where is the woman who was here?" I would, of course, say: "No, Carolyn, it was just you and me in this bed." More often than not she looked at me extremely quizzically as if to say, "Why do you say such weird stuff?" There frequently was bedding bunched up between our two bodies. She always covered herself with a sheet and with the quilt on top of our bed. I, on the other hand, used only the sheet for cover and lay my section of the quilt off to the side which was naturally between us. This bulk is what in the darkness of night resembled a body to her.

One early morning she became particularly irate with my denial of the presence of a woman. "I saw her arm around your face," she scolded, "don't tell me I imagined that!"

In the face of outbursts of anger such as that one, I learned more and more to stay relatively calm (and I do mean relatively) by centering myself. I would literally place my mind's focus at the base of my spinal column with the signal from my mind to my body: "Release all tension, let go of the physical strain by choosing to neither push nor pull anywhere in my body. Neither push nor pull anywhere in my body." I knew from years of practice that as soon as the physical tension leaves the muscles, tendons, and skin the body relaxes. The relaxing sensations, as simple as they are, go to that part of the brain where dopamine and endorphin are released, and immediately the mind is enjoying calmness, collectiveness, coolness - the opposite of uptightness, scattered-ness and hot-headedness. Why? Because those chemicals are hormones which give the feeling of well-being.

Obviously, I did not invent this marvelous technique which results in relaxation of body and calmness of mind. I had learned it from multiple sources and had taught it to my patients repeatedly over the course of my professional career as a psychotherapist.

My teaching the techniques which people used to acquire the skill included recording tapes in live relaxation sessions in my office. After patients laid back on the recliner provided and tried the techniques in a live session, I provided take-home tapes as reinforcement of the technique's steps. The instruction that went with the tapes was: the more frequently you practice the technique, the sooner you acquire the centering skill.

I knew from my own years of experience and by the abundance of positive feedback from many patients that this process worked because mind and body know, by nature, how to work together as one i.e., acting as one. And the more frequently that occurs, the greater the potentiality for success. This is especially useful when the human organism is under assault by real and imminent danger.

The successful athletes and warriors who manage to accomplish extraordinary feats under the most stressful and fearful environments are humans, like you or I, who know how one simple signal (from mind to body) can trigger the response from the entire organism to stay focused and to be able to go beyond boundaries in the face of all apparent odds. Like a football coach teaches: "You can hit harder than you can hit; you can run faster than you can run." And why? "Because," as another coach might tell us, completing that insight: "Your body can do things your mind does not know anything about."

I was and I am fortunate to have been a student and teacher of this process to de-stress the self and/or prevent fears from reaching panic or anxiety attack stage. In this sense, one of my prior careers had handsomely bestowed upon me something of tremendous and immeasurable value in order to be able to handle the multiple paradoxes presented by Carolyn's Alzheimer's disease.

And, to repeat, one of the major paradoxes was that she appeared so normal except in her inability to recognize me as her husband. She could recognize "his" picture and say to me, "That is Edward." She said it right in my presence as if she were talking to a new acquaintance. It was as if I were someone else to whom she was showing Edward's picture; it was a weird experience.

It became immediately evident in those first 19 months, when we were facing the new reality virtually alone, to retain and reinforce by all means much of the normal as possible.

She had quickly lost interest in cooking so I had to assume responsibility for what happened in the kitchen, obviously. Cooking was something Carolyn had done without a second thought for our 44 years of marriage. It became incumbent upon me to make plans for what we were going to eat. Not being a cook, I was limited to suggesting microwavable, pre-prepared foods. Fortunately there were many choices. By 2015 frozen, microwavable foods were fairly to very good.

It felt very normal and not risky at the start of our new reality for me to go to the grocery store and safely leave Carolyn at home. This simple activity of grocery shopping was just one more area of life which I needed to not just brush up on but learn to do. It had been her bailiwick for all our married life. Fortunately, because we had done many things together like this one, I had her imaginary footprints to follow. We had never been big on going out to dinner regularly. We'd go, but not habitually. It soon became habitual to go out just to get freshly prepared food. We liked the prepared frozen, but preferred the freshly cooked.

Carolyn had begun having a hard time relating to check writing, to understanding how a calendar works, how to read a menu, and how to read digital clocks, digitalized ovens, or microwave ovens.

She had resisted handing over to me paying of bills - a function she had jealously guarded since the first year of our marriage. Thing was she was forgetting how to fill in the lines for the checks. The many errors she was making caused many re-writes and tons of frustration and embarrassment for her. I finally managed to convince her that it was no big deal for her to allow me to assume that burden which she had carried all those years. I had been aware all that time of the truth in the axiom: "Who controls the money has the control." I did not mind letting her have this control because I had learned early in our marriage that, although I made better money than she did because of the inequality of how the genders are paid, she managed money better than I did. I never lived to regret that judgement, so she finally acquiesced and allowed me to take that monkey off her back. That was the beginning for me to start making major decisions about our life, hers in particular, without her input. Even now as of this writing nearly two years since she died, it is still a new sensation to be totally in control of all decisions about my life and the possessions which we amassed together.

One more area of life for me, one less for Carolyn.

Try as I might and did, I could not help her out of the cognitive dysfunction which made any normal monthly calendar a puzzle for her. She would ask questions about the calendar which I could not find an answer for. For instance, she would point to the Fridays (only the Fridays) and ask why they had lined them all one on top of the other: "Why?" she would ask. Or she would, with great impatience, ask why there were blank squares at the beginning of the month, (if that month's first date was a Monday or any other day but Sunday). Or ask why did they leave blank squares at the end of the month (if the month did not end on a Saturday). "Why?" she wanted to know.

My answers made so little sense to her understanding that she was convinced I didn't know either why they lined up the Fridays one on top of the other nor why there were blank squares at the beginning and end of the months on a printed calendar.

The problems with menus came about particularly once she developed lactose intolerance. She needed to see descriptions of food which told her what was safe for her to eat or avoid. The problem was compounded once the cognitive dysfunction became more and more pronounced. Because of this we went out less and less. There were too many choices on the menu and the lactose intolerance led to problems with eating sufficiently to maintain the appropriate calorie count and protein levels, etc. Carolyn lost so much weight due to poorer and poorer nutrition that her primary physician finally persuaded her to follow up on the referral to an endocrinologist who referred her to a nutrition specialist. This resulted in me counting calories for every item for every meal because she had an increasingly harder time wanting to eat anything but peanut butter and jelly sandwiches. More newness for both of us.

Carolyn had always watched her weight but she became scrupulous over a slight belly protrusion which she swore made her look fat. Had we not gone to the endocrinologist - who treated her with great respect - and the nutritionist, she might have gone to full blown Anorexia Nervosa. At five feet and three inches she carried 130 pounds well. She had sunk to 98 pounds. I felt like a failure for that decline.

Getting her to take in a minimum of 1500 calories daily became an ongoing hardship. The hardship for her was overcoming the fears of the anorexic. Fortunately, she liked the professionals helping her in this, so she avoided the extremes towards which she had been heading.

At this juncture of "Carolyn goes to retrogenesis," I want you to hear my journaling along this journey of Carolyn and myself.

This is a sample of some of my journaling. I did not journal daily. When I did at times my entry went on for several pages, like the following on July 25, 2012:

At 4:50 am Carolyn directed tremendous anger towards me as I awoke and walked out of the guest bedroom where I had slept that night. She approaches Ed with a flash light (not menacing in any way). As I was putting on my hearing aids and glasses and met her in the hallway. Angrily she asked and said at the same time 'That was not you in that bed?' and wanted to know 'Where he had gone?'

I simply replied - not reacting to the anger - that that had been me in that bed and that no one else was there. She yelled that there had been a boy and there was a man bigger than me in that bed. In her fury, she wanted to know why I was doing this to her.

She also expressed anger at another time because I had not slept in the same bed as her. When I explained that I had not wanted her to re-experience waking up in bed and believe there was a stranger there she ridiculed me for being such a liar because she had never had that experience, she insisted.

I did not contest the 'liar' accusation but felt it deeply.

I guided her to the kitchen to take her meds from kitchen cabinet. She followed without protest and did take the pills around 5 am. She had already fed our two cats.

The angry words and accusations of not loving her and being a liar resumed and continued back to the bedroom.

I said nothing.

She then ridiculed me for 'playing so innocently.' (sic)

We both crawled back in bed.

At 7 am I awoke her for her 7 am Namenda medication. She took it and was still seething with extreme anger.

I apologized sincerely for making the mistake of sleeping in another room. I admitted to her that that had been a serious judgement mistake of my part.

She did not say she accepted the apology but she didn't reject it either like she had when I first tried to apologize. She did change in mood and slowly became more positive.

I made remarks about the coffee. Small talk. I inquired of the head ache she had mentioned at 5 am. Gradually she talked more and more civilly.

By 9:30 am we had chatted. I had begun to iron clothes - hers first - she read some of the paper. She went and showered and emerged feeling much better she said.

By 11:30 am we ate lunch. I had continued ironing. We chatted while I ironed and she sat at the kitchen table. She asked about 'the other Ed' the one who had been a priest, 'where was he,' she wanted to know.

I casually responded, while ironing, that I was he. She then wanted to know whether if really, Alex and Moe were my brothers. I told her 'Yes and Bette in Las Vegas is my sister.' I had said that and she casually took in the information and quietly said she had a hard time associating me with them. She then wanted to know if I was the Ed who had lived in New Orleans.

This all transpired as if it is perfectly normal for us to be discussing two Ed's. At one point, she even laughed at our discussion and said she was going to have mark one Ed with a blue dot on the forehead and the other one with a black dot. That way she could differentiate.

We followed that conversation sitting in the T.V. room listening to music on our CD player. Some of what we conversed was her telling me things about her and Ed (the husband). She is talking very normally and casually not aware of the underlying reality that it was, of course, us she was telling me about. (I cannot exaggerate what a strange feeling it gives to have experiences such as these).

She suggested we go to Luby's for dinner, I enthusiastically endorsed the idea. She had recently talked to one of our neighbors who is a nutritionist and whom Carolyn loves and respects from her she picked up tips for regaining some of the lost weight. Now that she was at 97 lbs. she was a bit frightened.

Her cardiologist had suggested to her to take Ensure and her psychiatrist had added Boost to the suggestion. Unfortunately, both contain soy and she is highly allergic to soy.

After calling her nurse practitioner for a renewal of prescriptions, we changed after she had napped approximately 30 minutes. We were going to Luby's when she casually asked where the nice gentleman was, the one who had ironed all afternoon.

I played it down so as to not show my surprise and simply said that that had been me. Again, she replied she was going to have to mark me with a blue or black dot.

She proceeded to recount how nice that gentleman had been and told me what the neighbor nutritionist had recommended. By then I knew she had been with the non-husband Ed.

Her next question was: 'Where were you all day and what did you do?' She was cool with my response that I was the one ironing. I continuing believing that by bringing her back to the reality of my presence that something would click in her perception of me. Nothing did.

We had a quiet and pleasant wonderful dinner. We took some leftovers home. She fell asleep watching T.V. When she awoke and was going to change into nightclothes she asked if I were going to sleep here. I said yes which pleased her. She compliantly took the pills I handed her: cholesterol, Namenda, and Donaxapil.

When my narrative described this or that as having been "casual," I mean to stress that there was an absence of contentiousness in that remark or reaction where frequently, in our new circumstance, stress and strain had tainted much of our dialogue. It was wonderful when neither of us experienced the negativity in that. Like when I recorded that we had "a wonderful dinner at Luby's." What was wonderful was the ease with which we were both able to be living through a strangeness loaded with super hurt and able to suspend the hurtful through the grace of something of utter simplicity. We had what many "happy couples" have not yet experienced. It's easy to feel relaxation at a beach of white, white sand and quite another to feel at ease in the middle of a battlefield. (All analogies are limp, especially when one is looking for one to resemble Alzheimer's disease).

Once again, I choose to take the reading audience to more journal entries to demonstrate the context in which this whole narrative took place. I believe it's one thing to read a clinical report which, by definition, has a certain lack of the personal about it. It is quite another to feel the ground one is walking on and the wind blasts whipping the neck to and fro in a gale; with that, please see my witness of five pages of a journal entry on August 11, 2012 (three months since Capgras began):

This past week has been the longest episode of Capgras syndrome with her going day and night after day and night of inability to believe that I am the Edward she is missing.

In the first part of this week she had been amicable with the non-husband Edward but as the week went on she became first hostile to the non-husband and then increasingly angry towards the husband whom she now believes had summarily abandoned her.

She began telling the non-husband what a terrible person her husband was for his lack of respect for her and his lack of concern not only about her but about the house which she now has to manage by herself.

The more she stayed on these themes, the more she pronounced that she was through with her husband and did not want him back even if he returned. (The sting of this was severe to me).

She began making preliminary plans to divorce him because of all of these feelings provoked by his departure.

I tried to counsel her to 'Please let's first talk to (her psychiatrist) about these feelings before she approached any lawyer.' When she rejected that idea, I suggested 'Let's talk to the financial advisor (whom she respects enormously) before any more moves on the divorce front.'

(I had already alerted the financial advisor about the irrational behavior going on, in case it occurred to her to try to make some decisions about the finances we have).

When she rejected this idea, I argued for a discussion with her one in-town relative, the sister Lisa whom she has cherished dearly and always had since Lisa was a baby.

Much to my surprise she rejected these ideas as well. I finally went to suggesting Jan the one woman she had come to consider her best friend and whom she admires greatly.

She said no to that also. I tried not to sound alarmed.

All week she's gotten weaker physically and has become increasingly more teary emotionally with the anxiety triggered off by the mere thinking of these drastic options which she's been feeling compelled to take - all because she is feeling desperate, alone and uncertain about so much.

My quiet but persistent message has been 'I know you feel alone, but you are not, I am here. I never left.' Her answer: 'You are not the one I married.'

I feel that I need to feed my hope, that if I stay with this message, something will get triggered off to change her perception of my countenance.

No matter what I bring up about our marriage, that only she and her husband would know about, she finds a reason to discount it.

At one point, she looked at me almost with a compassionate look, 'I can't believe you because you want me to, not even just because I want to.'

This piece of clarity floored me.

What is keeping my hope alive in the face of my failures to 'trigger off' that desperately desired response is reminding myself of that reflex principle which I have placed great credence in 'for lo! These many years.'

The principle states that the history of life has born out repeatedly that 'every circumstance, every situation and every person contains its diametrically opposed side, i.e. everything contains its opposite and at some point, that opposite appears.'

In view of this assumption on my part, I see the principle of opposite to her disbelief, even if I do not know how to bring it about. I do not feel helpless when I tell myself that something in this universe, apart from me, can materialize the opposite of her disbelief.

CHAPTER SEVEN
THE RESPITE OF THE MOMENT

Today on August 11, 2012, we have had a giant of a marvelous breakthrough. After all of the talk about divorcing the "scoundrel husband," the one who obviously "does not love her," I started talking in almost hushed tones of my history with her. I brought up our first date and things about me when I was still active in the Catholic priesthood. I reminded Carolyn that because I had been tapped to become the Director of Charities for the El Paso, TX, diocese, I had wound up at Tulane pursuing a Masters in Social Work because I had been told by my diocese, "You don't need that degree, your office needs it." (Tulane University School of Social Work was where we had met.)

I went on to recount how she and I had met in New Orleans, the history we shared as students, who my friends were in graduate school, and who were her friends. I brought up the Mississippi girlfriend of hers who played Cupid for us and the summer we met in Dallas when she lived there in 1967 with her Dad and stepmother.

Carolyn picked up on the familiar imagery I was alluding to and the people in our first encounters.

Slowly, she began to cock her head, nodded in agreement in places of my streaming narrative, and, finally, she smiled with a glee that was muted at first and said: "So, you are the one who's been here all along!" And she asked as if the issue had never been brought up before which of course was precisely what I had repeatedly brought to the surface. Suddenly, her face lit up and it was evident she was seeing me in a new or different way; she was not talking to me as a recent acquaintance. She was talking to me as she did when she knew automatically that I was the one she had married years ago - 10 houses ago.

She recognized with clarity that she did not have to embark on a divorce! She realized that she was never left alone to fend for herself and her house. In one insight, she "saw" that all the strangers in her house - all the Edwards - were me! Had been all along! She was filled with a beautiful joy. She was radiant. I was ecstatic.

Before long we were hugging and kissing like two lost souls who had just found one another. Me as delighted and grateful for her awakening as she was with her new knowledge.

I saw, too, the disappearance of the fear she had expressed when she contemplated that some tragedy had befallen her husband.

I cannot express my joy that she was back. That something could "trigger off" a new way of perceiving me. And did!

I am not believing this was a miracle; I am believing this "opposite" ability of hers has been in there all along like all opposites are. It was granted to us that "opposites" emerge. Life does that kind of thing.

The following day saw a slight reversal of the breakthrough with Capgras; it wanted to rear its ugly head but barely could. It was gone and the breakthrough marshalled forth.

My journal entry of 18 days later notes that:

Last night marked what felt like a major crack in the breakthrough revelation of 8/11/12! Tonight before - right before - she turned over to sleep she tapped my shoulder and asked quietly 'Where is Eddie-Freddy?' Eddie-Freddy had been my nickname at the Florida vacations with her brother's family, Cookie, Ken, Eileen and Emily plus Cookie's sister Mary and her daughter Heather (cousin to Eileen and Emily). Her use of that nickname for me as her husband betrays tremendously pleasant and beautiful memories of past events in our marriage. It was a nickname that immediately brought a smile to my face corresponding to the smile on her face as she pronounced it playfully.

I responded, 'I am Eddie-Freddy.' She turned away, pulling the covers over her, saying: 'I was looking for the shorter version!'

No more was said.

Entry of journal on August 29, 2012:

This day at 7 AM she looked at me as I awoke and asked as if for the 1st time: 'Who are you?' She looked at me hard, quizzically. I said, 'Let me get up and put on my hearing aids and glasses and turn on some light.'

As soon as the light went on she beamed at me and exclaimed: 'It is you! You didn't look like yourself for a minute there.'

We hugged and kissed and laughed. I told her that I was afraid I had lost her. Her response was that she had been walking around the house looking for me and she didn't know who the strange man was in the bed.

By 9 AM we are still Capgras free. She confessed - almost sheepishly - that she first wondered who was in bed since 1 AM. And 3 AM. And 4 and 5 AM. During the whole time, she was experiencing Capgras in between spasmodic naps."

Journal entry on September 3, 2012:

From Aug 11, 2012, to now, there continues being an improved understanding of what constitutes Capgras for Carolyn. Up to this date, she had insisted that this syndrome is a condition imposed (given) to someone like her by a group of people such as the ones she believed she was talking to at a time, when all along, it was me she was talking to.

Now she is voicing credence that those 'people' were 'figments of her eyeballs' (sic). She can and does acknowledge that it has been really me - her husband - to whom she was talking.

She now expresses great delight to discover that she was not in fact abandoned by Edward her husband. It is remarkable, after all that we have been through, how clear all of this is to her. She wonders out loud what might have caused it. She no longer believes that I brought it upon her with a group of people trying to trick her. She now wonders whether someone, some unknown someone, 'experimented on her '(sic) to cause Capgras.

Today she slept three long naps. Highly unusual for her. One nap from 11 AM to approximately 12:10 PM, one from 11:20 PM to about 2:00 PM and a third one from 4:30 PM to 5:30 PM.

She then started falling asleep after dinner at 7:30 PM and went to bed by 8:00 PM.

Of great significance and concern to me is that between naps she admitted not only to fatigue and sluggishness, no-anti-anxiety meds in her system either - and, quietly without pronounced emotion, said: 'Maybe it is time for me to go to Assisted Living or to the funny farm.'

She has never voiced this in any of our conversations. She was serious when she said it but I could not detect whether she meant it seriously. My counter was that she does experience crisis sometimes, but most of the time we are both ok and not in need of anything other than our home right here.

I sincerely mean this and intend to keep her convinced of this - I do know, in the back of my mind, that eventually I may need staffs who can help her 24/7 but do not know exactly where nor when...

I have been feeling that everything weighs like a major struggle though Capgras is not the predominant condition now for 3 weeks and 3 days. This had lightened the burden considerably.

She has begun, once again, her volunteer work at the gift shop once a week and has now done if three Thursdays in a row. She has returned to attending the Monday morning breakfasts with girlfriends, Liz and Glee...admits to feeling somewhat awkward.

She has gone to lunches with friend, Jan Carter, every time she can which is absolutely great because no one energizes her like Jan Carter.

The weight problem has deteriorated considerably. Thanks to the suggestion of our neighbor who is a nutritionist, Carolyn has followed the referral by her Primary to go see an endocrinologist; she is to see a nutritionist referred by the endocrinologist tomorrow and to have blood drawn to determine further recommendation.

Her eating patterns are improving. She and I have worked hard to get away from the practice of constant peanut butter and jelly even if she was adding apple or banana to that diet. Now she is eating meals.

The lactose intolerance problem was so pronounced and causing her such frustration that it was in reaction to that that she became habituated to peanut butter and jelly. The habit is broken. She deserves much credit for this accomplishment. Indicates to me that she is dealing with the on-going frustration in less destructive reactions.

Whatever complexities may contribute to the practice of the disorder, Anorexia Nervosa, my observation of Carolyn is that she developed a fear to eat because lactose intolerance could make her severely ill if she ate the "wrong" thing. After a while the fear took a life of its own and eating became a problem whether she averted to the dangers endemic to lactose intolerance or not.

Her weight continues around 100 lbs. only, but fortunately the 97 lbs. low did not go lower before reversal began... still needs much reversing.

We are counting calories assiduously. Not because she tends to over-eat, obviously, but to counter under-eating... needs 1,500 calories at least.

It was beautiful music to my ears to hear her voicing 1st the experience of losing her husband but then her joy re-finding (sic) him and able to rekindle the marriage. The rekindling has been with affection and loving behaviors.

I too feel definitely like I lost her and then found her again or more precisely, have her again, because I never lost her, she lost me which is was why I couldn't have her.

There is a paradox somewhere in there.

Another measure of her improved condition: The medications and the dividers of the pill boxes are no longer the subject of the confusion which they had been, starting since early May 2012. Such a relief.

She is faithfully taking her 5 AM meds on her own without reminders. I do the reminding of the 7 AM and 7 PM Namenda medication - many 7 AMs and 7 PMs she is remembering on her own.

Planning future events still causes considerable consternation and anticipatory anxiety to the point where she plans poorly.

The calendar throws her off completely and because it does she is apprehensive relating to it.

CHAPTER EIGHT
THE CRUELTY OF THE MOMENT

For a good while, maybe twelve months since Capgras first appeared, we continued watching her favorite TV programs from 7:00 to 10:00 p.m. I usually watched 5:30 p.m. national news and 8:00 and 9:00 p.m. news channels. She rarely watched those. By approximately May of 2013 she was through watching TV; she would begin a program and in 5 to 10 minutes she would leave and go to get ready for bed.

We had without a spoken word worked out a very smooth pattern of each changing into our nightclothes separately in the bathroom, one following the other with no set determination as to who went first.

I would give her 20 to 30 minutes after she left the TV room and go in and say goodnight. If I was feeling like she was seeing me as her husband, I would give her a goodnight kiss and she would be receptive to that. I must have judged correctly because I never upset her with that affectionate display.

It was the same for when I came in from the store or the gym which I tried to maintain going to for no longer than one and two hours. I would gauge how she was seeing me to decide whether to do the goodbye or the greeting with a display of affection.

One time, I remember having totally misread the signals. We had gone to a pharmacy in a drugstore and we stood in line and I got right next to her. She quickly told me not to stand so close to her. "People will think you are my husband," she chided. It wasn't a harsh rebuke but it felt like a harsh rebuke. It took strength from somewhere to just maintain silence and obediently step back.

Carolyn had retired from Morningside Manor in 2010, but she continued going as a volunteer to help in the gift store from which she could go visit many senior citizens whom she had helped admit to the home. She usually went twice a week and thoroughly loved it. Prior to December 2012 she was able to drive herself there. This was one of those areas of normalcy in the midst of the abnormalcy of that period of time. Close to that December she told me with some concern in her voice, "For a while there, when I started heading back home, I had no idea where I was, but as I kept driving the road became more familiar again." As I say, she was concerned. I was alert as she recounted to me her lost feeling. I could not help but remember our major fiasco going to Montgomery the December before and how thoroughly lost she was back then.

I made it a point to drive her to her volunteer station from then on. She did not pick up on the fear I had of her becoming totally "disoriented as to place," and feeling totally alone. She accepted my offer to drive her to and from.

One scary night episode that same December 2012 resulted in her never driving again and it had nothing to do with driving.

She had been sound asleep and the same for me right next to her. She woke me up in a frightened state, telling me that she had been startled by a dream she had just had while half awake and half asleep: "I was staring straight ahead and I saw these bright lights spinning and spinning and they were many colors and they were beautiful but they were making me dizzy and I got scared and they finally stopped and I can still kind of see them." I immediately went to her side of the bed and helped her stand up. She kept saying, "I have to get my balance; that is why I need to stand up slowly and make sure my feet are planted firmly on the ground."

By the time she was standing up, I had turned on some light; she was almost giddy recounting how the lights kept swirling and how they were so beautiful and scary at the same time because she was getting so dizzy. Her giddiness continued until she was able to catch her breath and sit on the side of the bed, just taking in the emotionalism of what had just transpired. The strangeness of it did cause her anxiety level to rise, but there was an aspect about it that made her feel that, yeah, she had just experienced something truly out of this world and spectacular.

She spoke of the experience quite frequently with a certain glee and delight. For some time after that, she developed the anticipatory anxiety that the dizzying and spinning lights might appear while she was driving; this convinced her that it was not safe to drive.

I quietly believed she was doing "the right thing for the wrong reason" and did not argue the point. My anticipatory anxiety that she might get lost when alone was firmly in place. I was delighted that she did not want to be behind the wheel.

One event between her and her sister, Lisa, reinforced my theory that "disoriented as to place" was more of a probability than a mere possibility. As Alzheimer's became more pronounced, I witnessed the incremental but real progression of retrogenesis.

Her sister had taken her out shopping one Saturday as she and Carolyn had frequently done. These outings were a source of great socialization for the two of them. They thoroughly enjoyed each other's company and were champs at having a good time together. In this period of time when Carolyn noticed herself losing more and more ability to do simple, normal things, she looked forward with keener interest to being with Lisa.

Not only was she not driving to one of her favorite activities, the gift shop at Morningside, she had begun to lose interest in going to the gift shop. This was not because I was driving her but because the cash register (computerized as it was) became increasingly embarrassing and challenging. She began to avoid it and even fully avoided going near it. She had by that time made herself more homebound - not wanting to go to movies, not to grocery shopping, not to gym, not to visit friends. Lisa's apartment was the only visit she would not turn down. Going out for Saturday shopping with Lisa became highly important in the face of so much self-imposed reclusiveness.

Somewhere in the timeframe of the "shining and spinning episode," the two had gone to a rather large mall and, while in the department store Macy's, they became separated as frequently happened in their habitual pattern. They were used to going in different directions and then looking for one another before leaving a given department. They always managed to find each other again and again.

I later found out from Carolyn that she had suffered a major scare during this particular outing because Lisa had "abandoned" her and she had no idea what direction to go in to find her. This went on for she knew not how long, but it seemed interminable until finally she came upon Lisa accidentally.

Lisa had not abandoned her; she had done what they always did, knowing they would find each other again before leaving the department.

Carolyn lost her ability to follow the pattern of theirs, and neither she nor Lisa knew that Carolyn had already followed that particular pattern for the last time.

In this incident, Carolyn was in a totally unrecognizable situation, as if it were the first time, that she was alone without Lisa by her side. She panicked. Fortunately, Lisa came up to her before Carolyn acted out her panic. That convinced me that she was now in the realm of probability of getting lost if she were alone outside the home.

From that incident on she began to turn down Lisa's invitation to go shopping; feelings were understandably hurt on both sides.

CHAPTER NINE
THE TWISTS AND TURNS OF THE MOMENT

A third major event of December 2012 occurred - like the others - out of the blue. As I have said more than once, Capgras from its inception on that fateful May 12, 2012, had not been a permanent state. It came and it went with result as described up to now. Then at 1:00 to 2:30 in the morning a second awakening took place. She shook me awake, she turned on the lights, and she had a smile on her face; she had a look of happy surprise. She said, "I have been looking at you and I would see you, Edward, and then momentarily I would see a stranger, then you again and then the strange man. You have been here all along." She asked with the grin of someone very satisfied with herself, "You never went away, did you? You have been the one with me all along, haven't you?"

I was, to say the least, ecstatic!! I could not believe the revelation which truly had to have a divine origin. It was revealed to her by her experience of seeing me and the disappearance of me to her perception, and the reappearance, and the disappearance - all in front of her vision.

"My eyes have been deceiving me!" she proclaimed. "You never were gone!" With each repetition of the revelation, her jubilant mood increased as she was reaching magnificent crescendos at 2:45 in the morning in our bedroom. Both pairs of eyes danced in thanksgiving to God Almighty. Just as the saying goes: "There are no atheists in foxholes." There aren't any in such 2:45 a.m. revelations either.

It goes without saying that we could not contain our joy and genuine happiness. It would have constituted a major challenge for any third party to tell who, between the two of us, felt the more "found and lost no more." I truly felt as found as she did. She felt she found me after being lost in these strange roads and paths in the forest jungle of Alzheimer's which we were still euphemistically calling "cognitive dysfunction."

I felt "found" of course because, at last, her senses were not deceiving her that I was mysteriously absent. Her eyes found me where they had been seeing someone else taking my place.

My prayers of petition to the Creator of the Conscious Universe were immediately converted to prayers of thanksgiving to that Creator.

Our excitement lasted until probably about 4:30 a.m. when we finally were able to return to sleep.

The excitement continued the next day and the next for perhaps two weeks. She was able to recount with amazing detail to her psychiatrist, in my presence, exactly how and what was revealed to her; she saw nothing supernatural in any of it. She merely experienced the event as one where her eyes had momentarily quit seeing me and then could re-focus, as it were, and begin to see me clearly. We each reveled in the telling of it. So did the psychiatrist.

I could not help but notice that in this breakthrough, just as in the first one of four months prior, Carolyn saw herself as having been in Capgras due to an eye aberration. Neither time did she blame her mind when she saw someone else in my stead. It was her "eye balls" (sic) which were tricked. I did not bring any of this up to her.

That experience reached its apogee in about three weeks and then the revelation disappeared. Capgras returned to hold court until

May 2014 doing what it had done before coming and going with no particular rhyme or reason.

Like everything in the created universe, "It came but did not stay." And that was what I had to be conscious of in order to continue to experience the totality of it as part of how things are in life - for all of us, all of the time. It served to reinforce the whole outlook of living in the present, living in the moment; seeing the wisdom that instructs us to appreciate the imperfection of the moment, striving to comprehend the *Sacramento del momento* - the Sacrament of the moment - which reveals that in every happening the totality of the real presence is making the present possible precisely because the real presence is never absent as it is "the Presence without whom there is no present."[2]

That December we turned the corner of the first Christmas season in the land of retrogenesis. And, no, it was not the same, of course not. It was not cynicism to expect otherwise. It was being present to what circumstances life was presenting to us.

I decorated our beautiful home with the few Christmas decorations we had downsized to. She did her best to contribute to the preparations for Christmas. The minimal she did was treasured for the value she brought to "the doing." One simple example: I was putting tags on gifts which I had wrapped for nieces and she picked up a tag - which I still have - and wrote:

> *To Edward My beloved husband is so happy to help, Santa who will help me. Lots of love. I love you. Carolyn. Santa and I both know Edward is the best and the loving wife wants only the best for him and happy new year.*

(The grammar was poor. The emotion: beautiful).

------

[2] John Phillip Newell, *A New Harmony: The Spirit, The Earth, and The Human Soul,* (San Francisco: Jossey-Bass, 2011), xii.

Moments, like when she wrote that, peppered the canvas of struggle and strain with an easy flow of appreciating the beauty of the simple in life and the power in that simplicity - the eloquence of sincerity in whatever form.

We did little that Christmas. Opening presents seemed awkward to her. She didn't say that she felt awkward; she just acted that way. Going to Lisa's apartment was something she looked forward to doing. Once we were there, however, she acted out of step. I wasn't quite sure whether she was seeing me as her husband or not. She had quit being the Carolyn we knew, so she was not being herself with me. I could tell that she was also struggling to be and act normal with Lisa and Lisa's girlfriend who was there and whom we had both known for years. The gathering there was just for a visit and to exchange gifts; there was nothing formal about it.

When we left (she was glad I had picked up her signals for a "Let's go" without her having to say it out loud), she quizzed me about my familiarity with Lisa's friend who is a married woman. Carolyn felt that my normal friendliness was a bit much in light of the fact that I had barely met her. When I told her that, no, I had met that friend long ago through Lisa, Carolyn became momentarily lost and asked, "How long have you known Lisa?"

In that gathering, Lisa gave to me a present which had been given to her and which she knew she would not use - ever! It was a journal with a leather cover, one of the nicer ones. Her friend, who worked at the same place, had received a similar gift from their mutual employer. She, too, knew she would not journal, so she also handed me her handsome leather-bound journal. Tone of voice indicated quite strongly to me that Carolyn's complaint about my familiarity was really a complaint over the familiarity of Lisa's friend toward me. In Carolyn's mind it should have been clear to Lisa's friend that I was Carolyn's companion. She wanted to know, "Why did she give you that present?" All this conversation took place between Lisa's apartment and our car. Then I had my answer: Carolyn was seeing me as a companion; she was not seeing me as her husband. She did feel relieved when I pointed out to her that Lisa has known of my journaling habit for a long time and her girlfriend was just following her lead in order to get rid of a present which irritated her more than pleased her. Both Lisa and she had been upset with the boss for the Christmas present given to them.

Carolyn did not appreciate that friend flirting with her male companion! I have to confess: I felt a tinge of a thrill that I witnessed a spark of jealousy. At a level deeper than this ego-trip was the realization that sufficient bonding had been built up between Carolyn and the impostor in order to have meaningful trust in that relationship. Something we were both cooperating with was resulting in a positive in this thing from the dark side of life. I had lost my wife but was paradoxically her prime caregiver and she liked me. Who has that kind of good fortune? Those who believe that, indeed, "Nothing is too good to be true!" To paraphrase a modern aphorism.[3]

In this first phase of our new existence it was curious that she was failing to recognize only me. There had been moments when she started not recognizing her surroundings while driving back from the gift shop. It wasn't until later that I became aware that home began to appear strange to her. She "knew it was but did not feel it was," and she said it that way because apparently the strange feeling about home would come and then quickly dissipate. She'd stay with the recent memory that it had felt strange, but the feeling did not stay.

At times we'd be preparing to go to a given destination - a doctor's visit or a restaurant, something - and she would gather, say, a picture, some underwear, a book, or some such things and put them in a plastic bag. When I'd ask, "What are you doing, Carolyn?" (I

_____

[3] Kobi Yamada, *Ever Wonder? Ask Questions and Live into the Answers,* (Seattle: Compendium Publishing, 2001), 18.

would call her "Honey" if I was feeling like she knew me for who I was) her answer would be, "I am taking these things home." I had learned to not confront her with facts from my reality. I would not contest her. By the time we had gone to wherever we needed to go, the feeling of "this isn't home" had passed and approaching that subject served no purpose.

For a long time, I hoped that my reactions and the reasons that formed the basis of my reactions were at least okay, if not the best way to handle these situations. Many months later I received wonderful feedback in a training session for caregivers: it does not serve a useful purpose to address a banana with logic, because bananas, obviously, do not reason. Similarly, we were told not to use reason with someone who is acting irrationally because they cannot reason. I had thought I was on the right track, but I needed this consensual validation to be sure.

The allusion to the banana, at first blush, sounded almost insulting. I then remembered the anecdote about Coach Vince Lombardi's legendary insistence to "always remember the basics." To that end and while holding a football in front of proven professionals in the game, he would begin his season's training with the observation, "This is a football."[4]

The tenor of our life at 9106 Rustlers Creek, San Antonio, Texas, was pretty much what I have been describing well into the first five months of 2013. That made it just coincide with the first anniversary of living with what Capgras brought into our lives - May 2012 to May 2013.

---

[4] David Maraniss, *When Pride Still Mattered: A Life of Vince Lombardi,* (New York: Simon & Schuster 1999), 274.

CHAPTER TEN
THE PENDULUM SWINGS OF THE MOMENT

What changed dramatically in May 2013 was that Capgras became a permanent fixture in our existence. That is, from May 2013 until February 2014 - a full nine months later - Carolyn never again saw me as Edward her husband. The impostor in all "its" disguises became her ever-present companion. Ironically, because retrogenesis had had a year to gain some traction much of the anxiety of the first year subsided considerably.

From May 2013 on, one year since Capgras began, there appeared fewer signs that Carolyn recognized many familiar objects. Areas of decline which had popped up occasionally now began to appear with more regularity. For instance, whereas she had occasionally forgotten to take her morning or evening Namenda (for Alzheimer's), as 2013 wore on she forgot it more consistently and even reached the point where she did not remember that that was part of her treatment regimen. Consequently, she put up more of a fight as to why I was insisting that she take it. A similar thing happened with Donopazil, the other of her Alzheimer's medications. Activities which she had performed quite naturally now began to be tougher for her to see or recognize as part of her life. For instance, going to see her primary or her psychiatrist became fraught with excuses for not needing to go. She could not hold on to the positives of her relationship with her primary doctor. Evidence of this came in the form of suspicions about the doctor's motives for wanting to see her or for prescribing this and not that. Up to 2013, Carolyn idolized her primary and they had enjoyed a mutual respect for each other.

With time, Alzheimer's was taking the form of paranoia.

She lost all confidence with her psychiatrist after one session where he demonstrated impatience with her irrationality due to her full-blown Capgras. I was sitting adjacent to her on a couch in that session, as I did in all her sessions with him, and she denied having seen her husband for months. At this point the doctor impatiently blurted out at her that I, her husband, was right next to her and that, in so many words, she was putting me through a "rollercoaster" life. Paranoia had already begun affecting her opinion of him as well as of her primary. From then on she balked at going to see him even when she had forgotten the precipitating incident and, when he tried to add one more medication, she strenuously rejected his prescription.

The unfortunate consequence to that rejection resulted in her spurning an antipsychotic - Risperidone. I consulted with two psychiatrists who strongly believed that this drug might help Carolyn curtail the delusion which had her seeing impostors rather than me, her husband. Their judgement was based on the known experience with that particular medicine and how it deprived known psychotics of their known hallucinations.

At home, paranoia accounted for her distress over misplaced jewelry pieces which, time after time, she was unable to find. She had forgotten where she had hidden this jewelry and she angrily blamed "the loss" on "the others" whom she swore lived in the basement which we did not have. In her paranoia she never did resort to kicking or hitting as some do. She did some cursing, but that was negligible (and then it wasn't paranoia).

It wasn't long before the paranoia about lost/stolen jewelry spread to the conviction that clothes and pills were also being stolen by these intruders over whom she had no control. Because she feared they would perpetuate their behaviors again, she would stay in an angry state of mind for hours. That's where the cursing came in.

In this time frame, she imagined smudges on paintings or prints on our walls. To her the smudges represented the type of damage that changed the complexion of the content of the work of art. This understandably infuriated her and she looked to me, her companion - in one of my multiple forms - to ameliorate the situation.

I was totally helpless in knowing how to respond to this aberration of perception. To have denied the smudges (which of course did not exist) would have been tantamount to telling her she was wrong or silly for being as outraged as she was. That brought on the charge of not caring for her things as she did.

More and more, she was needing for me as companion or as Edward the husband - whomever she was perceiving (before May 2013) - to feel exactly as she was feeling about a given issue. If I didn't she took that as enemical.

Fortuitously, her anger would pass rather quickly because her recall of recent memories was increasingly harder for her to hold on to.

From May 2013 or there about, it was evident that Carolyn learned new information about anything less and less. There appeared a pronounced way of seeing life very simply. Thus, our everyday conversation became restricted to bare essentials. It was as if bright lights were turning to a soft glow. This constituted a quality of serenity amidst the turmoil brought on by all the changes going on in our life. Another paradox to behold.

She was managing to recognize friends and relatives other than me but had less interest or less energy in interacting with them. She felt an awkwardness in social situations which had never been there and which promoted more avoidance. This, of course, promoted more awkwardness due to increased social anxiety.

One of Carolyn's major forte's which had sculpted her into a better money manager than me - as I have alluded to above - had been her mental agility with numbers. In graduate school, she had breezed through research courses while I struggled for my "B" even with tutorial help to understand the abstract in numbers and statistics.

2013 saw her lose interest and ability to solve the simplest math, and when she did try, she never knew she had once known. This significant decline typified how we experienced her going away, slowly but surely. The Carolyn we had always known now manifested her inability to plan and/or organize social life, business concerns or health matters.

If Carolyn had been anything she had been a planner and an organizer!!

The tribute which I paid her in her obituary when I categorically stated that she won "Summa Cum Laude" evaluations in whatever position she executed due to the quality and quantity exhibited in her professional theory and practice was grounded in this mega-gift which she possessed. From her daily wardrobe to the efficiency with which she ran an admissions department, Carolyn planned and organized beautifully.

We made it to necessary meetings, with me doing the planning and organizing, and to doctors' visits or events with relatives and friends, even though it took an enormous amount of energy for both of us. Everything needed to be done slowly and with plenty of time and with kindness and patience because she was clearly more impaired than she had been in the prior 12 months.

I found it to take considerable strength to carry someone who had never required this level of care because it hurt so much to realize that this was not only a chronic condition of a formerly well put-together person but a condition destined to worsen in the fairly close future. The hurt lingered.

In spite of protestations which Carolyn exhibited more frequently and with greater intensity, she did take the prescribed Alzheimer's medications along with those for cholesterol and high blood pressure and thyroid condition 93% to 95% of the time in this period of decline. This alone demonstrated that with solid effort the difficult could still get accomplished by seeking alternate ways of doing things. One other upside to this life of increased simplicity manifested itself precisely in her enjoying the simplest of things and not demanding much out of life.

She would arise between 7:00 and 8:00 a.m., bathe and groom herself with fresh clothes and slowly eat simple meals. She would lie down once or twice in the morning - a practice she had never engaged in before - and then would attempt to read out of a favorite book of recent interest on the culture and spirituality of Native Americans. I say "attempt" because she could not read more than a few pages before she would put the book aside and tell me that she was going to talk to the Creator. With that, she would go to the TV room and sit on a chair which afforded her the view of our backyard's trees, bushes, birds, sky and clouds. She did her talking to the Creator alone and out loud.

I would be in the kitchen writing or reading the current events and could barely make out the sounds of a very sincere person talking without guile to a trusted and respected person.

From childhood, she had cultivated a love of nature and grew up loving all that breathes - from humans to the animal and vegetable kingdoms. She found a kinship in the Native American spirituality which sees spirit permeating all that exists. That spirit was the one she addressed as her Creator. Her theology was fiercely simple and profound to the core of her being. It was moving to be in the kitchen feeling the energy she was generating, evoking, and invoking. The air of quiet solemnity surrounded this home-spun ritual - all Carolyn.

Talk about an uplifting experience amidst such confusing newness. It was another paradox to behold.

In the afternoon she could take as many as three short naps - some very short - but these rests managed to pull her through what, at times, seemed like such a slow day with little to do. Carolyn's activity, though little, was extremely tiring.

For a prolonged period of time, from May to December in 2013, she could enjoy the afternoon TV show *Ellen*. Her affect was becoming more and more blunted but she seemed to enjoy the depiction of people laughing or applauding or expressing joy with one another. It was as if it pleased her to be in the presence of pleasing emotions even though she herself expressed fewer of these emotions. Had she been depressed I doubt she would have sought out the program *Ellen*.

Time came when this interest, too, went the way of the wayward wind. It was perhaps four weeks past May 2013 - like June or early July - that I began realizing that Capgras was a permanent state. There had been no natural reversals and certainty no more breakthroughs like the ones we experienced in 2012.

Carolyn was not aware that the husband Edward was not appearing anymore until approximately September of 2013. By then it had been four months that Capgras was in a permanent state and all she had encountered were impostors. Good to be able to report that, in this time period, the encounters were extremely positive with the non-husband Edward.

This state of things developed or unfolded to "a stranger than a strange" event; the experience emerged without fanfare just like Carolyn's first break with our reality unfolded when she first was the victim of Capgras and I, as her husband, suddenly disappeared.

It began to dawn on Carolyn that her husband had not appeared in forever (I say forever because she had long ago been unable to relate to divisions of time which we call days, weeks, months or years, yet she apparently could perceive when a long time was a long time). She started remarking how Edward had not been around in such a long time and that perhaps, this time, he was never coming back.

She said this enough times to come to accept her observation as a fact.

At first, she began quizzing the non-husband if he knew where the husband was. She seemed to have the impression that it was usual for non-husband to be able to connect with her husband. She showed signs of knowing that somehow this Edward who could pass for a brother to her husband was connected to the husband in some strange way. She would express mild surprise when she was told that "no," non-husband was not in verbal contact with the missing husband. Oddly enough, at these times, Carolyn did not express anger towards the missing husband whom she suspected was communicating with people around her.

It was as if this oddity was unchallenging to her any more than we are able to challenge the incongruent elements which we experience when we are in the land of surrealism dreaming away in subconsciousness - pardon the redundancy.

As days and weeks wore on with these realizations about husband's absence she began to ask whether she and non-husband could marry.

WOW!!

She had long ago dropped talk of divorce. Now she was not even seeing that as a necessary step prior to another marriage. She made it clearer and clearer that she wanted to know whether non-husband was willing to consider that option of marriage since they were always together and "just to make things right."

There had been no other preliminaries to this wish for marriage. No talk of love or forever... just whether I, non-husband, was willing to marry.

WOW! I was not expecting this thunderbolt of a proposal. And once again I immediately intuited that I dare not show shock or any emotion that could hurt her feelings or seem to put her in a negative light. I reacted as if that were a normal option for "us" to consider.

Internally two opposing and powerful emotions were absorbing my attention. First, a deep sadness immediately hit me that she was ready to disregard me, Edward, her husband from her life because she was actively believing that I was being so cruel, so insensitive, so non-loving, and totally disrespectful by staying away from her for so long. I was totally helpless in assuaging this feeling of hers.

Secondly and simultaneously, I was feeling joy without bounds for being selected, again in my lifetime, by the woman I most loved, to be her husband. For a lifetime.

Both emotions overwhelmed me.

I dared show only the latter emotion. Immediately, without hesitation, I gave her assurances that, yes, of course we could do that and did not need anyone's permission. In the same immediacy, I imagined a simple ritual - homemade - right there in front of our fireplace with a few friends and relatives. I told her of my image and she liked it. She liked it a lot. That pleased her.

I was careful not to make any commitment as to "how soon" or "how far off." I intuited that I could forestall such a move if necessary so that something sacred did not turn into a farce or something that could cause derision.

It pleased her immensely that her wish was grantable. The positive mood which this evoked lasted a considerable amount of time. Two or three days would qualify as "considerable" for one with a shorter and shorter memory of recent events.

She returned to this theme several times at two or three week intervals and, when she did, it was as if we had never discussed it before. The positive in that repetition was that it brought new joy every time. And, no, we never did have to nail down a time as to when it would happen. As I said earlier, she did not relate to the future as she had prior to retrogenesis. She just couldn't.

My enthusiasm at her requested wish was genuine because I chose to focus on the positive emotion of being selected again.

The longer time elapsed from May 2013, when I last remembered her recognizing me as her husband, the more this wish of hers faded from the reality she was in. By November or December of that year, the subject of marriage evaporated completely. It felt like an evaporation.

We had long ago discontinued going to the gym together, since perhaps October 2012 or approximately five months since Capgras made its entrance. I had continued going perhaps two to three times a week by myself until approximately May 2013 - one year after Capgras.

We had continued our routine walks in the neighborhood - walks of one or two miles - all up to November or December of 2013. Whether lack of interest or tiredness, something just prevented this activity from being part of our routine. I realized later that there had been a hint of a lack of interest in our neighborhood and I could not help but wonder whether that neighborhood had begun to look unfamiliar to her. To this day I do not know for sure.

What I did know was that "home" was becoming more of a prominent obsession. "Take me home," or "When are you going to take me home?" or "Why won't you take me home?" or "Please take me home!" All of these questions arose when we could be in any one room of our home or at any time of the day. Rarely at night. Not all four questions came at once. These were the many ways she had begun to demonstrate that not only did she not identify with home as a familiar place - our home of 28 years - she was showing, with out being able to articulate it, that she was feeling unsafe where she was. She was seeking safety and security of environment. She was in fear.

I have mentioned earlier in the narrative about this journey to retrogenesis that Carolyn would pack some items as we prepared to go to a given appointment and that I would inquire why she was taking those things such as underwear or pictures or a book, etc. Speaking of whatever she packed in plastic bags, she would answer that she was taking these home. When she began doing this she had not prefaced it with an explanation that she didn't recognize our surroundings as her home. This became evident through her behavior and her subsequent reasons for those behaviors. (It was as if she thought that I knew that "this" was not our home, so there was no need for her to tell me so.)

I did not contest anything in these instances. I merely helped her carry out her preparations by placing her bags - never much in them - in the backseat of her Nissan which I drove all the time I took her places.

At those times we would go to our appointed round and return with the plastic bags - by now forgotten by her - still in the backseat of the Nissan.

Later, when she wasn't looking, I would return the items to their corresponding place in the house.

At this stage of her retrogenesis her desire to go "home" became pronounced in the manner of the questions she was now asking.

When this manner of questioning arose, I detected that she really meant for me to quit stalling and "really, really" take her home. What I did on at least four occasions was to say: "Ok, Carolyn, let's go see if we can find your home."

I had known for a prolonged period of time that she was dealing with me as if I were the trusted companion who did everything Edward had done - and more!

We would then get in the car - with her happy as a child going to a candy store and me determined to go 20 blocks if needed - and I would engage her in conversation about this landscape or that tree or who lived where and when was it was that she last saw so and so, etc., etc., etc. These simple conversations were sufficient to get her neural pathways onto other interests and distract her from searching for her house/home.

Often times four to six blocks were all that was needed and I knew I could take us back home because her desire of wanting or needing to be elsewhere was gone. She would be okay on this subject for two or three days.

On one of these jaunts of searching for home, we had gone eight or nine blocks from our address and were in a very different looking part of our neighborhood. Suddenly, she bolted upright and pointed at a house we had once identified as a possible residence for her dad and with great joy and satisfaction screamed with glee, "There! There it is!"

She was at the height of purely positive excitement and there was no way I was going to contradict her "find" and spoil her exquisite delight, so I said as I slowly drove past the house, "We'll have to go back for the key. I didn't bring the keys!" I then asked her whether she had the keys and, of course, she said no, so I repeated what I had said and by then we were blocks away from the "find." I said, "not to worry" and that, first, we needed to go get the key. With that she was able to hold on to her emotional high until it came down of its own accord.

I drove to no place in particular for perhaps 20 minutes and when the conversation about the house died down I was able to drive us back home without incident. She never brought it up again and neither did I.

To this day, four years since that momentously joyous event, I can vividly remember and re-experience the sheer delight and joy she emoted when we arrived upon what I have since denominated as a vortex of powerful and superior energies - all positive, all straight from the magnanimity of the Conscious Universe - to bring happiness to a person who had had her share of suffering major uncertainties and their consequent fears and horrors. The re-experiencing occurs when I drive by that exact location. I drive by there at least five times a week. It always makes me smile to remember her smile. The "re-experiencing" means I do not just remember that joy, I re-live it.

CHAPTER ELEVEN
THE EVOLUTIONARY LEAP OF THE MOMENT

It took some time for me to reach the realization that not recognizing home carried the element of fear more and more.

At first I responded to her "take me home" with the rational approach to something which was not a problem of reason. I softly but firmly insisted: "But Carolyn, this is home."

Never had I read or heard that Alzheimer's patients "wander off" due to fear of where they are. I always assumed they wander off because they are confused.

Confusion may trigger this response, but I thought upon reflection of Carolyn's pleas that I detected anxiety over not knowing where she was and anxiety is another name for fear. In the state of anxiety one is seeking to fight or to flee because of a present or anticipated danger or the perception of such.

When the reason behind this obsession became more clear to me, my alarm buttons sounded ferociously that "I need to make life safer for her."

Up to that time I was subconsciously looking to the medical profession for guidance. I expected her doctors to clue me in as to when the time would come to place her in one of those sanctuaries called nursing home, or assisted living, or psychiatric unit. Not only "when" but "which" of those would be indicated and by what omen(s)?

I truly had no clear and distinct idea how to handle the next inevitable waterfall in this river of life which was sweeping us along. And we used to think we were in control!

When she began telling me: "If you do not take me home, I am going to call the police, or a taxi, or I am going by myself," it was at that point I realized her genuine fear. I took her fear as the omen I had needed as to "when" to find her a better sanctuary than what I could provide. At home she was now a flight-risk.

I immediately began to explore assisted living and memory care facilities. Carolyn's sister, Lisa, and I put together a list and the two of us began to tour and interview four such facilities.

The one we both agreed upon was an assisted living facility specializing in memory care for Alzheimer's patients.

During this period of searching for a place for Carolyn, the theme that kept running through the back of my mind like background music centered on the question of how had it come to pass that my wife of 44 years would now have a more complete life if she had three shifts every 24 hours because she was no longer safe at our home and simply could not take care of herself. I knew, too, that finding an assisted living facility for Carolyn that specialized in memory care for Alzheimer's patients meant she would never return home. She and I would be separated permanently. True, we no longer had the normal married life we had enjoyed prior to Capgras in 2012, but we had been geographically close, day in and day out, living together even in a fairly intense set of circumstances. Now we would be together no more, and Carolyn did not even know it nor could she know the intense pain this caused me and how it affected all who loved her. We all knew this change represented a totally different trajectory for us which had no "u" turn.

We soon discovered that our search was taking us to the harsh reality - harsh but necessary - that these sanctuaries have locked-down units for those considered flight risks. The lock-down feature is there because some residents in need of assisted living are Alzheimer's disease patients, so there exists an understandable segregation built in which isolates the flight risks from those who may not even suffer Dementia. Many in assisted living are in Dementia. Many are not. My wife was. I was no longer calling it cognitive dysfunction, but Dementia.

In my psychotherapy practice I had done a considerable amount of in-patient work with psychiatric patients from 1982 to 1998. The in-patient part of my practice was all in lock-down psychiatric units so the locked-down feature in itself was not a shock to me as it naturally is to many family members when they first see their loved one behind locked doors.

What did shock me to the core was the extremely crowded conditions which the at-risk population appeared to be in within in these otherwise fairly spacious assisted living facilities. Another s-h-o-c-k to my senses was how much more disturbed those Alzheimer's patients seemed in comparison to those who were roaming around in spacious spaces.

One group looked like the senior citizens they were, all with varying degrees of disability due to the old age we are all headed towards if we are among the chosen who get to "the evening of life" - as one colleague taught me to regard old age.

The other group resembled thrown away lives in bodies beyond frailty or in wheelchairs which were hardly moved. This group resembled the shuffling wounded whom the non-sensitive mental health workers used to cruelly refer to as "those with the Thorazine shuffle" (Thorazine being one of the first anti-psychotic medications).

Carolyn was, by this time, a flight risk but by no stretch of the imagination was she ready for a motionless wheelchair or an environment devoid of stimulation. She was not to be grouped with anything thrown away.

She had declined on the retrogenesis chart to Stage 4 with one feature of Stage 5 "needs help to remain safe in home." She did not always act like an 8 to 12-year-old as the chart ascribes to those in Stage 4.

One significant drawback that I see in the retrogenesis chart in relation to its presentation of certain characteristics assigned to a developmental age is that one could conclude that a person with those characteristics at that stage is always at that corresponding age level. That was not the case in my experience with Carolyn.

In my experience with her Alzheimer's journey, Carolyn developed the characteristics assigned to the various stages, but she did not always act at the age assigned to that stage. She would dip into that age level more and more as she exhibited particular characteristics but the dip was always from a higher age bracket. Much like when we hit 13 years of age, we do not immediately behave all the time like an adolescent of 13. Some time after that 13th birthday we might revert to the behaviors of an 11 or 12-year-old or we might demonstrate the behaviors of a 14-year-old. But mostly we act 13. The behaviors of the 13-year-old become more and more prevalent, all things being equal, until we hit age 14. The same patterned phenomenon occurs when we hit 14. Again, we are not immediately one year older in our perception or our comportment. A similar pattern existed for Carolyn, but in reverse.

The assisted living memory care for Alzheimer's patients that we picked for Carolyn was one totally locked-down and not just in one segregated area. The place is so constructed that a long and high wall enclosed a vast area around two-thirds of the back of the entire facility. In that enclosed outdoor area one can walk extensively, as if in a half moon, from one end to the other. There exists 30 to 40 feet of grassed-in area replete with trees and shrubs and flowers, picnic tables, chairs, barbecue pit, and benches all accessible to the entire patient population via six or eight exits or entrances.

The doors are electronically opened at a given early morning hour and locked at a given nightly hour after supper. The patients and their guests can come and go in and out all day or can stay indoors in activity rooms provided for activities and visits.

Here, Carolyn, who loved to walk, had ready outdoor access whether alone or with whomever was visiting her.

The place is so constructed that two CNA's in tandem with an on-duty nurse care for 16 patients - a desirable ratio.

At full capacity the place holds 64 residents and groups them into what they denominate as four houses. One "house" is at each corner of the central complex.

Each house consists of a complex of 16 rooms - all private. There is one kitchen and a dining room for 16 dining guests, laundry facilities for 16, and entrances and exits at two ends. There is also a recreation room in each house with a huge TV and easy furniture all around.

The facility provides medical and dental specialists or allows families to take their beloved to outside professionals.

Aside from the positives of the physical layout, all the services which our long-term care insurance paid for were provided.

We were fortunate that Carolyn had had the foresight 17 years prior to the onset of Alzheimer's to acquire long-term care insurance, so we were in a position to afford the expense which all this entailed.

Another recurrent theme underlying all this planning was the long-held assumption that, since I was nine years older than Carolyn, I would go first. She and I never said it out loud but we both knew that we both knew that this was just the logical thing to expect.

Never had it crossed my mind that I would be in the role of her primary caregiver and, ultimately, the one to find a place for her outside of our home.

I had read the book and seen the movie *Still Alice*, as I have alluded to earlier in this narrative, and I had no idea that I would have the role Alice's husband had to assume.

What that story prepared me for was the built-in frustration for the medical profession. There is so little research on Alzheimer's that not too much is known that can give much hope or guidance. There are medications which are purported to halt the progression, but the amount of guarantee is close to zero; "halt" is a very relative concept.

I say this because this info did not make me bitter. Frustrated, yes, but not over the top surprised that answers or predictions were few and far between.

The name of the new "home" we found for Carolyn was (and is as of this writing) Arden Courts Memory Care for Alzheimer's patients.

I made application for Carolyn to go on their waiting list in January 2014.

It felt wonderful to have found a place where there is no such thing as warehousing of senior citizens. We had found a place where she had no access to dangerous city streets (for one who has no sense of direction) and marvelous access to a very inviting outdoors space. Like many other places we had toured, Arden Courts provided a host of activities designed to be appropriate stimulation of the senses and of the mind.

After enrolling Carolyn for residency, I found it would be a waiting game until a vacancy opened up for her to be able to move in.

I had already communicated the family's intention that Carolyn be put on the anti-psychotic, Risperidone, because this drug would likely disrupt her delusions just as it would hallucinations. The psychiatrist there agreed to this request.

The Admissions Director of Arden Courts, who had known Carolyn in her position as Admissions Director at Morningside, suggested that I place Carolyn in a psychiatric unit to start her on that desired medication while we waited for an opening at the assisted living facility. This woman, who had admired Carolyn as a role model when she worked in admissions for Morningside, was providing me with guidance and information to help me find a psychiatric unit specifically designed for Alzheimer's patients. Before Carolyn moved in Arden Courts was already providing guidance for me through its director of admissions.

This was a tremendous revelation to find that a psychiatric unit was available to receive and treat Alzheimer's patients because, in my days as a professional in mental health, psychiatric units denied access to Alzheimer's cases. Psychiatric units, like hospitals, exist to provide curative care and, since Alzheimer's was incurable (even at the time of this writing), those facilities have been traditionally reserved for patients who had a chance of getting better.

This was another reminder of the cruelty of what my wife had inherited from both sides of her family - Alzheimer's disease.

Now knowledgeable of such a place, I began what seemed like a process of a 1,000 steps. I would sneak to our backyard and communicate by cellphone with an admissions nurse who listened to the particulars of Carolyn's case: diagnosis, by whom, when, meds, names of prominent doctors, presenting symptoms, etc.

I cannot put into words how treacherous it felt to sneak around in back (with her cell phone) in order to make arrangements to place her in a psychiatric unit - the type of which I had been used to going to in order to treat deranged minds in human beings who were at the mercy of others for their wellbeing.

The admissions nurse would take down the clinical information I was conveying and assure me that she would present it to two psychiatrists running the unit. From them she would get back to me for further information or clarification of what they already had been presented. At one point in these, what seemed like 1,000 steps, the nurse expressed the psychiatrists' doubts about Carolyn's admissibility as a candidate for their program. I re-presented Carolyn's pertinent symptoms, especially highlighting her flight-risk indicators.

Finally, they gave me the green light with a major caveat: since it was highly unlikely that Carolyn would enter their locked-down program willingly, I would have to get a court commitment.

Those words had the force of icicles piercing my heart, but I knew (what they callously call) "the drill." Here again, I felt myself, Carolyn's husband, "going through the drill" which would lock her up. Never mind that it was all for her own good. Of course, it was for her own good, but it still felt like imposing a sentence on a wife I loved dearly - "more dearly than the spoken word can tell."[5]

---

[5] Roger Whittaker, "The Last Farewell," *The Last Farewell and Other Hits*, RCA, CD.

"Court commitment" to me, from my past acquaintance with that procedure, meant a courtroom and a judge listening to witnesses of medical competence declare why a person needed to go to a psychiatric unit until medical professionals gave permission for release. That, in a nutshell, composed my mental picture of what Carolyn was going to go through, and I had no idea how we would put together all steps necessary for that to come about.

I trusted the admissions nurse when she assured me that all that would be explained to me at the right time.

I fought the image that crept up in my head of two burly cops forcibly escorting Carolyn to a court room. I did not know how but I vowed to myself that I would do whatever I had to in order to prevent her from being treated as my anticipatory anxiety was imagining her treatment.

When all was arranged for her to be admitted there, I told Carolyn: "Tomorrow I will take you home, Carolyn." By this time I had relied on the kindness of her sister, Lisa, and her good friend, Liz, and arranged for them to meet us at our home by 10:00 a.m. on the day of February 13, 2014. The psychiatric unit had instructed me to have Carolyn at the admissions office by 11:00. And, once we were there, admissions personnel would call the psychiatric unit and arrange for the court commitment there at the admissions office. I did not understand how that could be because I was stuck with my mental picture of a courtroom and a judge in a black robe and all downtown!

My recollection of patients going through admission to a psychiatric unit informed me, that from 11:00 a.m. to Noon, all would be said and done especially since the unit psychiatrists were the ones to be doing the pre-arranged admission.

I knew exactly where to go to a hospital no more than four miles from our home. Santa Rosa had four locations and one of their giant ones was close by.

When Liz and Lisa showed up at our home that morning, I matter-of-factly told Carolyn that they were to go with us to take her home. She was fine and happy with that. She was taking the move home quite calmly and with obvious, if not boisterous, joy.

Liz had arrived first and, in no time, was sitting quietly with Carolyn in our living room making small talk. Lisa had mistakenly gone to the wrong Santa Rosa - the downtown main hospital which does not have the psychiatric unit that we needed. Her late arrival did not complicate anything and gave Liz a chance to ease Carolyn into what the three of us intended to do with as much grace and naturalness as we could.

As we drove to the admission entrance, I asked Liz if she would park the car for us so that I could walk Carolyn in.

As I climbed out and went to open the car door for Carolyn, she registered a perplexed look and got out of the car asking, "What's this!" I quickly told her: "Honey, now that we are here why don't we have that stomach problem you have had checked out?" "They can do it as soon as we go in." Lisa offered her assurances that all was fine and that it was good that we were there. This helped Carolyn to feel more settled.

Between the three of us we kept assuring Carolyn that this was going to be a good thing to do. Her resistance was mild at first.

The admission procedure lasted from 11:00 a.m. to 4:00 p.m. Because Carolyn was being admitted to one unit of the hospital, she had to undergo all the testing required of anybody entering that facility. That included a social history, lab work (with time needed to get results back), x-rays for contagious diseases, etc., etc., etc.

All the information that I had fed to the unit admissions nurse had to be repeated again and some of it more than once depending upon which department of the admissions department was doing their piece of the entire process.

While this all took place, we were with Carolyn in a special waiting room within the admissions office. She was in a wheelchair and we sat with her in between the times she was taken to different hospital sections for the various components of the evaluation procedure. After each component Carolyn would be wheeled back to the waiting room to await the next evaluator to come for her.

Needless to say, this whole five hour chunk of time caused considerable stress and strain. It took the three of us using our wits and our imagination to prevent Carolyn from bolting from those surroundings. She wanted to know what we wanted to know: "Was all this necessary?" and "When was it going to end?"

We were tired, poorly fed, looking for answers and trying to sound like all this was normal so that Carolyn wouldn't blow the gasket which we felt like blowing.

Just when I thought we'd be there all night, a police officer stepped in the waiting room and quietly invited me to follow him outside of that room which I did.

He had me identify myself as the husband of Sara Carolyn Alderette. Then, very politely and with great courtesy, he asked me to given him a summation for the request for Carolyn my wife to be committed for treatment at that hospital's psychiatric unit for Alzheimer's patients.

I enumerated her symptoms and behaviors in summary fashion; I told him of the treatment she had received and from which doctors and gave the reasons she was a flight risk and why I could not contain her safely by myself and how she needed one medication to be administered in an in-patient unit because she would not take it on an outpatient basis.

He informed me that he would convey all this information to a judge who was standing by (through prior arrangement with the psychiatric unit) and that he, the officer, would get back to me.

He left and I reported to Lisa and Liz the latest development. Within 30 to 45 minutes the officer returned with two staff persons from the psychiatric unit and informed us that the judge had ordered the commitment.

The two staffers wheeled Carolyn to the unit with us following. There was not one single burly cop in sight.

The final step had been so gracefully and respectfully accomplished. Someone, times no-telling how many, had put together a wonderfully easy procedure to set in motion a necessary but hard commitment process.

CHAPTER TWELVE
THE MOMENTOUSNESS OF THE MOMENT

I was 80 years old when I engaged in this commitment of my wife to a psychiatric hospital unit. In my 80 years, I had seen parents - either the father or the mother or both but mostly the mother - suffer extremely when a first-born, particularly, "went off to college" for the first time. The "going off" apparently carried meaning on many levels and most of them were excruciatingly painful. Only another parent who had experienced such an event could probably appreciate the exquisite incision this event could have as it pierced the heart of the wounded parent.

In a similar way, except 1,000 times more, was the pain I experienced when my actions were calibrated to institutionalize my wife, if only for a short period of time, in a psychiatric unit.

There were, indeed, many levels of meaning in what I did and, with grace from my Higher Power, I was able to find one salient meaning which, like a paradigm shift, served to enable me to live with myself.

I had the presence to capture some of those levels of meaning in a three-page free-verse piece which I wrote and sent to as many people whom I knew who cherished Carolyn and loved her.

NO DRUM ROLL HEARD.
NO MUSIC OF TRIUMPH

NOR OF DIRGE TONES;
NO TRUMPET FLOURISHES
NOR FLOURISHES OF ANY NOTE
ANYWHERE
YET, TODAY,
A MOMENTOUS AND INFINITE SERIES
OF CAUSES CAME TOGETHER
IN ONE FOCAL POINT TO RESULT
IN THE COMMITMENT
OF MY WIFE TO A PSYCH. UNIT
BY ME
HER HUSBAND OF 46 YEARS.
I HAD THE HELP OF TWO WONDERFUL WOMEN.
ME, WHO USED TO BELIEVE
THAT LOSING ONE'S MIND
HAD TO BE THE ABSOLUTE WORST CURSE, EVER.

TURNS OUT IT'S NEITHER: ABSOLUTE, IN ANY SENSE,
: NOR WORST,
: NOR A CURSE.

IT'S AN EFFECT
OF AN INFINITE SERIES OF CAUSES
NONE OF WHICH INVOLVE: DISGRACE
:DISHONOR
: NOR DISRESPECT TO
LIFE

IT IS AN EVENT IN THE COURSE OF A LIVING PERSON'S
PATH THROUGH THE CYCLE OF LIFE
WHICH CAN CULMINATE
IN A TRANSFORMATION TO ANOTHER ENERGY FIELD
WHOSE FREQUENCIES
WE ARE NOT EQUIPPED TO PROCESS WITH
UNDERSTANDING,
MUCH LESS QUALIFIED

TO JUDGE AS A CURSE.
IT'S A TRANSFORMATION LIKE THE ONE WHICH WE,
NIGHTLY, GO INTO
WHEN WE ENTER THE WORLD OF THE SURREAL
WHERE LOGIC AND RATIONALITY,
INDUCTION AND DEDUCTION,
REASON AND ALL FORM OF SYLLOGISMS
GIVE INTO FANTASY OF THE BEAUTIFUL ILK OR THE
FRIGHTFUL AND TERRIFYING
WHICH WE CALL NIGHT MARE-ISH,
BUT NEVER A CURSE
AND CERTAINLY, NEVER, ABSOLUTE IN ANY SENSE.

WE RECOGNIZE OF THE SURREAL
THAT JUST LIKE EVERY SOLITARY THING ELSE,
IT CONTAINS ITS EXACT OPPOSITE
WHICH TAKES US
TO TAKE THIS AS AN OMEN
THAT THE LOSING OF A MIND
IS A STATE
WHICH THE FORCES OF THE CONSCIOUS UNIVERSE
KNOW HOW TO "BALANCE OUT"
FOR THE RHYTHM OF THAT STATE
TO FIND AND JOIN THE DANCE OF
THE ULTIMATE REALITY i.e., CONSCIOUS UNIVERSE.

COMMITMENT TO A PSYCH. UNIT THUS BECOMES
A PATH TO THAT "BALANCING OUT."

My commentary on the free verse:

You will notice that I began the free verse with an awareness that nothing in external reality announced what to me, to us, to Carolyn was a momentous undertaking. In the course of human events that event was neither victorious, nor dire, nor did it call attention to itself in any way, but it was such that it took an infinite series of causes to bring it about. Just like the production of this book in your hands required an infinite series of causes - going back to Mr. Gutenberg himself - and just like the rest of reality's web in which "anything" is connected to "every thing," it takes an infinite series of causes to be what it is. I am saying this event was special - just like all the other ones being brought about.

I then identify the immediate protagonists: the wife, me, the two wonderful women.

I allude to a belief which I once harbored about lost minds, a euphemism for psychotics, and how I had relegated that (them) to the bins of 'absolute' and 'worst' and 'cursed.'

I then summarily pull these last three from their assigned bins and declare that I now have evidence that a "lost mind" is not an absolute state nor in any sense in the category of worst and by no stretch of the imagination is it in the genus of the cursed.

I proceed to portray the causes which were calibrated to bring it about (the losing of a mind) as neither disgraceful nor dishonorable nor disrespectful of life, implying that if the causes were not so characterized so, too, neither is the consequent effect of those causes and the effect, I intimate, was the lost mind of Carolyn.

I then put what happened in the genre of transformation - not merely a change but a change upwards is implied - and the upwardness is to "an energy field" that enjoys frequencies vibrating above our pay grade.

I take the reader (listener?) into what kind of transformation is this upward change and I equate it to one of our most common experiences, namely, us in the state of dreaming while asleep.

I make reference to what is commonly experienced by all who remember their dreams when awake and aware that what we dreamed followed no logical sequence and that the dream world can transport us to actually experience beautiful fantastic feelings or of the horrifying stuff of nightmares. But, while in that state, we also realize later that nothing of absolute nature transpired, no matter how bizarre, nor did anything of a curse arise, no matter how frightening.

I then express (reveal) a level of meaning that had eluded me all the while in which I worked in psychiatric units with what I had considered awakened compassion for those whom I helped to treat i.e., those in some form of psychosis. I make note of the reality that in our experience of the dual world in which we live, we experience that everything exists on a continuum where everything then contains its opposite. In the dual world of materiality we see that the hot can be the cold, the here becomes a there, a strong can become the weak; the sweet, the sour; the good, the bad; the bright, the dull; the light, the dark, etc. etc. etc. ad infinitum. So too, I see that "the losing of a mind" has its opposite. But I conclude that "forces of the conscious universe" can extract the opposite of that, just as another vitality awakens my vitality. I come back from the surreal land where logic and its syllogisms do not exist to return to my world of materiality and join the dance of the conscious universe. I then formulate a new belief that the one who has lost the mind will also join the conscious universe and will do so through forces whose understanding is above my pay grade.

This significant level of meaning comes to me from the insight that commitment to a psychiatric unit is a path to the mystery we are all headed towards. The path we can see. The mystery, like all mystery, eludes us.

End of commentary

I definitely had a paradigm shift which enabled me to see Carolyn's state of mind as a reality different than the one I was encountering and the one we used to share.

It humbled me to admit I did not understand the reality she was in but I did not have to understand it to be able to accept it. It was incumbent upon me to respect the reality she was in and in no way be dismissive of what she was experiencing, no matter how bizarre. I was not to belittle that plane of existence she was in nor tolerate any one making fun of her "antics."

I did not have to become a preacher to others about the given insight I had arrived upon. It quietly instructed me that she was not to be pitied or relegated to being lost. She might be lost in our reality but she was not lost in the world of her reality. She was no more lost than we are when in we find ourselves dreaming and experiencing contradictory elements as if they were one.

Of immediate consequence to this: I found more and more reason to be as present as I could every time I was with Carolyn so as to be conscious of being responsive to her communications in word or action.

Her word was, from here on in, less and less intelligible. But there continued to be nuance in her voice and inflections and pauses to her speech. This flow indicated a message in transition and that message seemed to convey various moods or attitudinal adjustments as to what she was perceiving and attempting to give voice and expression to.

When I say I needed to be responsive, I simply mean it was possible to pick up on her intonations with sounds of assent or words of encouragement or simple acknowledgement that I had heard.

We might not have been on the exact same wavelength but she was not alone. An example: shortly after arriving at the psychiatric unit with people specifically trained to deal with this Dementia, Alzheimer's, Carolyn and a fellow patient would be in one or the other's room gazing fixedly at a minute section of a small pattern on a blanket. They were studying it as if they were counting the threads (or something even smaller) and making the slightest of slow motions with their fingers over the surface of what they were examining as if through a microscope. The small sounds they made were utterances of wonder and surprise. My reaction of presence to their present (whatever it might have been) was to simply and quietly say: "Glad you are finding such beauty in what you're finding. It's wonderful what nature reveals to us when we look closely." The moment taught me to stand there silently with her while she admired that pattern.

At first Carolyn would want to leave the unit when her visitor, whether it was me or someone else, needed to depart. But she never went into kicking or screaming at not being allowed to leave. (Some do. Her stepfather did.)

She was still bathing herself and able to select the clothes she wanted to put on. All this she did by herself. She was fully ambulatory. Shortly after her arrival there I noticed her new pattern of taking things like picture frames apart. I had brought framed pictures from our home for her to continue seeing familiar faces. She would pull plants or flowers out of their water environment. She worked on dismantling drawers in night stands, taking them out and attempting to unscrew pulls or knobs. She placed the drawers under the bed.

She walked the circular corridors and visited one new friend frequently. The point being, unless she was napping, she was mobile and not alone in her room. Staff reported how compliant she was in talking her medications, eating when fed, and retiring to bed when it was so indicated.

She did start the Risperdone and shortly began, for the first time in nine months of Capgras, to see me as her husband. By this time close to 20 months had elapsed since she began to lose major abilities. Some effects of Capgras may have been present, but there was now no big smile of surprise for my "return" nor were there recriminations for having "disappeared." There were no more reports of the others who claimed they, too, were Edward.

She had no recall of what experiencing Capgras had been like. She just didn't have any knowledge of what had transpired at our home for 19 months prior to this hospitalization nor of the admissions process she had recently experienced. The memory slate was almost clean.

It was as if we admitted her at precisely the same time that she was going through a major retrogenesis digression.

The fear she had begun to feel at home seemed to be the first warning of this major regression. Was she feeling the regression itself? I do not believe so.

It quickly became glaringly apparent that if Arden Courts had no room when the psychiatric unit was ready to discharge her (normal stay is no longer than 14 days), I would have to find a temporary facility which took her symptoms into account - particularly her flight risk.

The regression evident in 14 days was dramatic. Now she knew me, but now it was much harder to know her. One thing was certain: she now needed help in three shifts a day, 24/7.

Carolyn was at the psychiatric unit at Santa Rosa for 17 days - under extremely competent professional personal care. Unfortunately, Arden Courts was not in a position to accept her when the psychiatric unit could hold her no longer.

Hurriedly, I found what I believed to be ranked as a good nursing home. In my naiveté, I judged the facility by its open unit rather than its locked-down unit and made arrangements for her transport from the psychiatric unit to there.

I had had confidence to transport her from home to the psychiatric unit but now, 17 days later, I had no confidence in my competence to move her from there to the nursing home. Not even with the help of a willing sister and friend. I had checked out the recommended nursing home but had not even averted to the possibility that she would wind up in the closed unit. What I had seen of the closed unit, when I checked it out, was similar to what I had observed in the disappointing assisted living facilities with closed, lock-down quarters that offered no outdoor provisions.

The transport by professionals went fine with no resistance on Carolyn's part. I was there to greet her when she arrived.

Within hours of being in the open unit and all settled in, she was escorted to the locked ward because, as soon as I left, she inquired as to where the doors were which led to the outside. They knew better than to take a chance. Quickly, before I returned for the evening visit, they placed her behind the locked doors.

What existed behind those locked doors totally opposed the environment in which I had enrolled her.

I felt downtrodden. The closed unit, locked-down ward at this nursing home was a limited indoor space with no access to outdoors. It housed approximately 82 patients who were all flight risks and all in some degree of psychosis. Some seemed under chemical restraint.

One central nurses' station was headquarters for five to six CNA's who were there to attend to the population of at least 82 patients. To the right and to the left of that station sprang two corridors each of which contained doors to private or semi-private rooms.

The room assigned to Carolyn resembled a clean but nevertheless third rate motel room with very used worn out furniture:

one closet, one single bed, one night stand, one chest of drawers, a chair, no wall hangings, broken blinds on sealed windows, and one bathroom. One could pay for a decent-sized TV.

I am going on with this description to possibly ward off a major shock for some future caregiver who might be as naïve as I had been for not asking more questions.

The nurses' station was at the head of a rather large room - 30 ft by 30 ft - large enough to house six rows of tables and benches for perhaps 12 persons per row. There were no chairs; it was picnic-style seating.

This was the dayroom for the 82 and it became the mess hall at meal time. Besides their rooms this was the only other room available to the patients who had all day to kill - everyday.

The five or six CNA's were forever busy. They were either at the computer, dispensing medications or assigning meds to individual pill boxes, or picking up or delivering laundry to patient rooms. At mealtime, some swept while others distributed or picked.

I was there three times a day for two-hour visits in the morning, in the afternoon, and at night before bedtime. In those 11 days that Carolyn was there, I saw that those CNA's had little to no time to spend with those enclosed patients. And I saw that many of these patients never received visitors.

Those CNA's - all women of good nature - worked long and hard, but had hardly any time for "one on one." I could not fault them for placing Carolyn where she would be safe from the danger of running off.

What I could do was visit her three times a day to assuage any feelings of abandonment to a jungle of aimless human beings walking as if disowned.

By mid-March this painful stretch of road ended and she was taken by ambulance to Arden Courts.

Now she was in brighter atmosphere. It was a place where we the family had a choice of retaining the furniture provided by them or substituting any or all of that with our own furniture.

Their furniture consisted of a beautiful blond oak bed, night stand, closet, and chair, plus beautiful drapery and shades.

We had permission to decorate the walls with as much as we chose to resemble home, and their handymen did all the hangings according to our specifications.

Now she was in a place where she had six exits/entrances to and from a huge outdoor space. All enclosed by a high wall which concealed a beautifully landscaped area that was inviting to guests be they relatives or friends.

Not only were the CNA's at this place available for our input and to answer questions about our loved one, we had access to the personal attention of the director herself. And the admissions director had already given me tremendous encouragement by way of tons of information. I elected to have Carolyn transferred to the medical staff of Arden Courts, including the in-house psychiatrist, and the nurses who supervised the CNA's. All staff were personally available to us.

Another significant feature of the place we selected was that it incorporated, in its philosophy of care, to be as attentive to the needs of the respective caregivers of the people who had become their patients as well as to the needs of the patients themselves.

Arden Courts provided one-on-one ongoing support and information to caregivers, all in an extremely friendly and professional manner. One eight-week extensive program based on a workbook they provide is designed as stress-busting program for family caregivers. That is the title of the workbook which serves as syllabus for the course. It is a work of 174 pages consisting of nine chapters - all on the subject of a path to wellness and tailored to the role of caregiving.

The workbook is copyrighted by Sharon Lewis, RN, Phd, FANN who authored it with four other Phd's, two of whom are also RN's, one M.R.A. one B.B.A. and one M.S.T.O.M. One of these professionals is also a L.P.C and marriage counselor. (The work is worth looking up for any caregiver of a Dementia patient.)

In my opinion, every one of the nine chapters contains highly relevant information and insights for all caregivers - especially for primary caregivers who by definition carry the heaviest weightiness of the caregiving role.

The course was presented didactically and experientially. The depth of the experience came in the experiential component. This was a professionally presented training experience not just an educational experience.

We, the 17 or 18 regular attendees, received the opportunity to bond as a quasi-community for this part of or our caregiving journey.

After the formal course ended, seven or eight of us continued meeting on our own for monthly follow-ups for maybe six months just to give and receive additional support.

Facilitators for the course included the Director of Arden Courts herself, which redounded to her knowing us up close and personal - a plus for our loved one who was their patient.

My prior psychotherapy experience had introduced me to many of the topics covered, but many of those topics and themes are unknown in depth by the average lay person.

But even for me as an ex-psychotherapist (retired for four years at that time), it did not hurt one bit to rearrange old knowledge in my own makeup and to glean new insight (as the proverb instructs: "one can gain new realizations from ancient truths.")

Carolyn had not reacted negatively to the nursing home she had just left in spite of the fact that we, the family and friends, saw the place as dim, dingy, and impersonal. It seemed more like a warehouse for bodies who walk, yet there were exceptions to this. Like the three times in 11 days when a physical education tech came and took Carolyn out of her locked quarters and gave her one-on-one personal attention for 45 minutes to an hour.

Her reaction was one of docility and compliance. "Acceptance" might be too strong of a word. That docility was part of the new Carolyn we were witnessing emerge.

That same attitude and demeanor she took to Arden Courts from the beginning.

I quickly made it a point to decorate her room with as many furnishings as were appropriate for the size of the space. I decorated the main wall with a unique mirror and a brightly colored wall tapestry which she had picked out herself in Peru. I brought three of her grandmother's quilts, which she had displayed beautifully in our guest bedroom, to hang upon the wall facing her bed. I brought her English writing table (the very first antique we ever purchased 46 years prior) to hold a TV set and family pictures. Also decorating our guest bedroom back home were stuffed animals and toys from childhood which one aunt had thoughtfully saved for her. These, too, came to Arden Courts to grace one of the walls on a shelf which came with the room. The last two items from home included the black leather recliner which we both loved to sit in, one colorful rug for the area next to her bed, plus her beloved orange leather chair - a Queen Ann.

I detail all of this to highlight the urgency I was feeling - and was not even aware of it at the time - to bring "home" to her since this place, as far as I could foresee, was going to be her final home. When she had gone to the psychiatric unit and even to the nursing home I knew those were only to be temporary homes away from home. But this one, I knew, was to be for the forever which she would have on this earth. The depths and heights of that realization are beyond any words I can come up with. I desperately felt, "since she cannot ever be close to what home is, I need for some of home to be close to her so that she can continue experiencing the people whom home represents."

I wanted her to be touched - even if only in the gentlest of ways - by the anniversary related to that mirror, by the wonderful trip related to that tapestry, by the grandmothers related to those quilts, by the joy of a newly married couple related to that antique table, by her sis, Lisa who had given the TV set, and of course by the people who loved her in all the pictures on the writing table and the night stand.

From the beginning of this fork which the road took, Carolyn seemed like one who intuited the insight of some sage who tells us that in our waking state it is not life that we experience, it is what of life we focus on which determines our experience.

If she perceived any negatives they were few and far between. For instance, we began taking walks every time I would see her in the morning and afternoon. On these walks we would go in the directions of her choice. We always encountered others - patients and caregivers or other visitors or staffers going in the opposite direction. I would invariably greet passersby. Whenever we crossed paths with one particular patient who always walked briskly and alone and without a smile, Carolyn would tug at my shirt and warn me not to even look at her and to stay closer to our side of the walkway because she was a mean person who liked to fight. I never did find out what she based that judgement on. I simply did what Carolyn said as we walked past the woman - who, by the way, did not look mean to me. Our walks and that lady's walks were long enough that sometimes we crossed paths two or three times. Carolyn tugged every time.

Our walks usually started indoors and we had any of four directions we could embark on.

Indoors consisted of one central location which was surrounded by four corridors. In that center were housed the nurses' station, restrooms for visitors, hair salon, recreation quarters for staff off duty or on break, equipment rooms, two large rooms for patient activities or presentations to patients and/or their guests, and the central kitchen where all meals were prepared and carried to the four house kitchens.

One corridor led to a sub-complex called the green house - all woodwork including doors was painted in muted green. Green house consisted of a corridor of its own in an "L" shape with 16 rooms all total, off of the sides of its own "L" shaped corridor. At the juncture where the halls of the green house met, there stood a small kitchen complete with stove, refrigerator, dishwasher, and dish cabinets. Off of this kitchen stood a small dining room for 16 resident chairs. This dining room featured a door to the outside area which any one could go out of or enter through. Next to the dining room was a good-sized recreation room with a large TV set at one wall, one large sofa, and five or six lounge chairs.

A similar pattern existed at three other sub-complexes off of the central location. What existed for the green house existed for a blue house, for a red house, and for a yellow house. Color distinguished each house. Color made it easier for residents to find their rooms.

Each house was home to 16 patients. All patients who were ambulatory had access to the four houses.

Thus, anyone could go from one house to any of the other three because the four sub-complexes all connected to the central main complex. Also, one could exit or enter to and from the outdoors via any of the four houses.

Most of the walks which Carolyn and I took daily, at least twice a day, took the path of one house after the other. Each saw greetings to Carolyn from staff at all four houses. When I wasn't there, she frequented the three houses apart from the green where her room was and, by the account of the staffers who knew her the best, her favorite house to visit was the the blue house. Months later she would confide in me that the blue house reminded her of her dear Morningside Manor where she had both worked and volunteered for a huge meaningful part of her life.

After we visited the houses at least once, we would then walk the entire length of the backyard at least once, and frequently back again. At times we would sit at one of the three alcoves along the four indoor corridors surrounding the central location. Each had easy furniture. Or we would sit outside on benches and chairs located in various areas with various sceneries to enjoy. From the central area two exits took one to the outside or took one back indoors, as well as each of the four houses.

It may seem like I cannot stress enough how much this physical layout impressed me, and this is true. I cannot stress sufficiently how beautifully this layout served my Carolyn and by extension, us her visitors, in her 10 months stay there.

She came here immediately following a sizable decline in ability and in mental health status scale. She was destined to go down further because that is what Alzheimer's does.

This environment facilitated a gentle, kind slope. It allowed Carolyn to move downward into retrogenesis with grace, surrounded by an environment which cradled her. As she laid to rest more and more capacities, she remained safe in the doing of it all.

We the relatives and friends had the code to the necessary doors which allowed us to visit at any time without having to go through unnecessary screens each time.

The standing attitude of staff always welcomed us to inquire about any outstanding occurrence requiring our attention or to report to them observations which we needed to call to their attention.

From March 2014 to July 2014 - four months at Arden Courts - I made it a point to visit her three times daily during which we began the visit with walks as I have alluded to. In those walks I had a chance to be a visiting husband to her and to react to her communications. Her expression in language lacked more and more intelligibility but her tone of voice, her emotion as she talked, her facial expressions and other body language all spoke volumes. From those, I took my cues on how to react just like we react to a child who cannot communicate with words. This does not mean reacting with baby talk - which babies don't need either - but with some sound on my part which connoted my listening to her and my gladness that she expressed her feelings. Sometimes, of course, I had no idea how to react because the signals I picked up seemed beyond my imagination to comprehend, in which case I would usually just say "hum!" with the added emphasis of the eyebrows going up.

Priceless! When in the midst of meaningless chatter out would come a full sentence, clear as a bell, like "Here, we go left," as we approached a fork in the outside sidewalk, or "That is what we had for lunch," pointing to a printed daily menu hanging near the green house dining room. There was also, like I said earlier, "Don't look at this one coming. Stay on this side. She likes to fight," when we encountered one particular woman on our walks. Much earlier than this time at Arden Courts, Carolyn had floored me when, in the midst of a Capgras discussion, she asked, "Are you having a mental problem?" "I am not!"

When I arrived for a visit, I frequently had to go chase her down because she never stayed in her room. I was told by the staff there that she exercised her mobility constantly. I always knew to check out the blue house first and, true to form, I would often find her there.

In those first four months of her stay there, we had a ritual which entailed us imitating a TV commercial where boy meets girl out in an open field. As soon as they spot each other, both run towards the other beaming with outstretched arms and meet with a climactic embrace. We would mimic the running towards each other - usually started by me as soon as I spotted her. I would exaggeratedly throw my arms up as I went to her. She would imitate my arm flinging, and we would embrace with a smile if not a laugh. Then we would walk off holding hands. If there were onlookers, staff, or other residents, we would accept/acknowledge their faux applause and genuine smiles. We always walked holding hands.

The ritual meant the world to me because it genuinely pleased me to see her and made me enormously glad to see that the simple ritual evoked such a positive response from her.

I cannot remember what clue I received after about four months of doing this that told me, point blank, she did not know (anymore) how to participate in this simple display we had invented for the wonderful amount of time that it lasted. The ritual came to an end like every thing in transient existence.

We still had the foot rub custom. That did not change. From the very first, when we finished the afternoon walk and the evening visit, we would sit on the edge of her bed doing small talk. When it was close to going-home time, I developed the habit of leaning over her lap and gently picking up her legs so that she would be reclining on the bed while I moved standing up at the foot of the bed and proceed to remove her shoes. Then I would begin a foot rub, a massage to her feet which went to her ankles and the calves and back of the knees only. I never (deliberately) went higher than the back of her knees so as to keep it all strictly in the massage genre of activity and nothing sexual in the slightest.

I never considered it fair for me to initiate anything sexual with Carolyn because of her impairment. I sensed that I never would know her capacity for full consent once Capgras entered our lives. Even at home, for the 19 months after Capgras, I could not go beyond kissing her with no foreplay. The kissing became spasmodic pecks when she became more ill simply because of the possibility that at any unknown time she could revert into the Capgras syndrome. I did not want to be attempting to kiss her while she believed I was non-husband Edward (I could not even calculate the degree of confusion which that would have caused with the multiple impostors she had been experiencing).

In the Glen Campbell TV show of his Alzheimer's progression, someone indicated that the libido change cranked up quite high for the Alzheimer's patient.

I only experienced that with Carolyn one time; on one particular celebration of my return as her husband, she became quite amorous as a normal wife would. I let her take the lead in that one and all was fine with no incident of ill consequence.

I believe a spouse who is primary caregiver needs to be attentive and not cause added confusion for the Alzheimer's patient in the whole area of sex. In my case, as I have indicated, because

Carolyn believed she had to deal with more than one non-husband Edward I never ventured to introduce sex into that already entangled web.

And, so, I never did. I'm extremely glad because I cannot help but believe that, in Carolyn's case, sex would have introduced a set of complications that would have hurt a person already experiencing a host of hurts.

In my role as caregiver, I took seriously the effort to help avoid as much added confusion of the maddening kind as possible. I did not, under any circumstance, want to add to it.

My foot and lower leg massage would immediately result in the closing of Carolyn's eyes. In fact, she closed her eyes as soon as I removed her shoes. She never once objected to this custom.

I usually hummed love songs or tunes from a musical with which we were both familiar to her. I enjoyed my own humming and massaging almost as much as her peaceful look suggested she enjoyed it. Invariably, sleep overtook Carolyn within 10 to 15 minutes of rubbing and humming.

I never closed the door to her room while I performed this customary ritual. This meant that the outside noises of voices and doors banging and machinery whirring all entered her room but did not stop her from dozing off.

Romantics label these moments tender. To me, they expressed that and more. Every single time, these became living moments of profound awareness. I was so fortunate to be able to bring such peacefulness to my wife who was becoming sicker with a lethal disease inch by inch with every beat of her heart - and mine. Amidst the chaos in our lives and in the eye of that maelstrom came a magnificent peace to both of us - twice a day, seven days a week. A profound peace!

Once she was asleep, I would stay with her 15 or 20 minutes, just humming and watching her sleep (like she knew someone close was taking care of her).

By this time in her journey, well into 2014, she no longer feared abandonment. Carolyn had no need for talk of divorce or concern for who entered or exited her life. She responded *con gusto* to our rituals and customs which became part of who we were for each other. No words of mine could describe what couldn't be described anyway.

It frequently crossed my mind that, on the path to losing each other, we had so much more than many couples who were also just that year, just like us, past their 46th wedding anniversary.

At Arden Courts it became easier for friends to drop by. At times they found her sound asleep as I did on occasion or they asked staff to look for her in one of the houses. Visitors of course noticed Carolyn's decline since early 2014. They turned their visits into opportunities to demonstrate genuine compassion and acceptance of her condition. No one complained because they could not decipher her thoughts through the jumbled-up words and phrases. I gleaned all of this in my conversations with those friends when I visited with them.

I always believed that those visits, by all those wonderful friends, had tremendous meaning in that they served to keep a constant reminder for Carolyn that she mattered dearly to many. There continued to be an importance to her person which many wanted to and did acknowledge.

I wanted to believe that, in some slight but real way, all this seemed to register for our Carolyn, even in her poor comprehension of most of our reality.

I thought I detected a reaction by her to those visits (when we spoke of them) as the unspoken feeling of one who was aware of attention given - much like young children respond to adult attention in a matter-of-factly thankful way.

That was how I saw her react with Arden Courts staff who paid a lot of playful, loving attention to her.

I witnessed this same attention from the staff of the four houses which Carolyn frequented.

I say this deliberately because I know of the oft-stated cynicism that all institutions which provide care for disabled senior citizens treat every one as an institutionalized commodity.

Many exceptions exist to that type of behavior, and, certainly, Arden Courts was and is one just as surely as Carolyn's beloved Morningside Manor was and is as of this writing.

One month before taking Carolyn to Arden Courts I described her condition in a January 14, 2014, letter which I copied and mailed to 29 family members and friends:

Dear _____,

Please be patient with me as I try to succinctly and coherently give you a set of facts related to Carolyn's and my state of affairs.

Emotions, pros, cons, causes, effects and projections, all will be addressed at another time; here, just major facts for the sake of brevity - but hopefully enough to shed some light.

Exactly one year and eight months to the day of when Carolyn exhibited the first major symptom of what was later diagnosed: A brain pattern consistent with Alzheimer's disease, on 01/18/14 I moved to place Carolyn's name on a waiting list for an assisted living facility which specializes in the memory care of men and women who are in need of intense memory care for Alzheimer's disease. Intense meaning the need to receive care in an in-patient setting so that it can be consistent, on-going, 24/7 with three shifts daily of professionally trained people.

You may remember, she first experienced Capgras on 5/12/12… that syndrome came and went.

In the last 20 months (1 yr, 8 mos) she has seen me as her husband, maybe 5 months of that time-period.

*In the other 15 months, she has seen me as "a friend."
A new friend who at first was a total stranger.*

The last time she knew me as her husband was May 2, 2013. She was awash with joy and jubilation for about 17 days. Then I disappeared again to her.

To assuage her suspicion, or anger, or hostility to me, the stranger, my role has been to make myself indispensable by simply doing all that Edward did and more, that is, with loving compassion, with nurturance and affection. Being the human whom she is, even in illness, she has responded to me positively even if with a question mark.

Her strong belief is still that Edward chose to abandon her but that he is still around, though he does not show his face to her. She believes others may see him. It is as if she senses his presence, though she does not see him and believes others may see him. The progression of the cognitive dysfunction is now such that I can no longer be her sole provider.

She needs more stimulation than the company of one friend. She needs the structure in life which she once knew how to organize and effectuate. More and more basics of life loom into becoming major mysteries; like how to regulate hot and cold water in a shower, or how to tie a shoe lace, or write a check or what are the steps to making up the bed? Or how do we find the house?

She misses people, she yearns for the family she had when she belonged to Morningside Manor - (her employment for the last 10 years of her work outside the home). Her anxiety is more frequent and intense and it lasts longer.

More paranoia is evident, more fears of being vulnerable to "them" who have already stolen clothes, jewelry or changed her clothes or down-sized her jewelry. Is fatigued with more regularity. Finds less interest in T.V., in reading, in exercising, in eating.

She will be at Arden Courts on Huebner - about 15 minutes from where we live, as soon as an opening comes - could be 3 to 4 months. Maybe less. Probably not longer.

I will address the selling of the house... as soon as this dust settles from this current turbulence.

I will give more information as weeks take us deeper in this forest - uncharted by me - for sure!!

> *Love You*
> *Thank you for caring,*
> *Please continue the*
> *requests from the Creator*

CHAPTER THIRTEEN
THE METAPHORS OF THE MOMENT

The metaphor of the forest keeps surfacing in my subconsciousness, to give a visual of what this journey - another ubiquitous metaphor - looks like. Forests replete with known roads and paths are one thing; uncharted ones, presage only the unknown to the right, to the left, forward, and behind.

Up until the writing of this letter I had barely become accustomed to one set of patterns in Carolyn's behavior when gradually, (which felt like suddenly and, paradoxically, suddenly felt like gradually) her behaviors changed to another type because her skill set diminished as the days of the year ebbed.

The rate of change was truly incremental; meaning of course, it was so slow it was almost imperceptible to the senses of the body. Yet the change appeared like a flower suddenly blossoming when, all along, it has been coming to a ripe stage.

I believe that when people say things like: "I didn't know whether I was coming or going," they have experienced what I am talking about here.

At times like these I took it as an omen that the time had arrived when I needed to take a timeout from the world in order to practice more mindfulness. A mindfulness process with its centering essence awakens me to slow down sufficiently to be able to distinguish the simple in "suddenly" and the simple in "gradually" as well as the understanding of the trajectory of "coming" versus "going."

I think it is called "getting one's bearings." Then I realized: "Carolyn cannot, any longer, get her bearings." That realization saddened me greatly and signaled, clearly, one more reminder to be compassionate with love as well as protectiveness.

This made me recall the poetry and art of Brian Andreas who has written:

> *My calendar makes it look*
> *like I have everything*
> *under control…but I ignore it*
> *& treat every new day like*
> *the emergency it is.*[6]

The full force of the insight in the last sentence hit me like a double thunderbolt when I realized that what I had been going through with Carolyn for 19 months at our home was: "Each day an emergency."

Interestingly, that poet Andreas in his knowledgeability of the human psyche is really saying (in my interpretation) that, whether or not we know it or whether or not we are in a predicament such as the one which Capgras subsumes people into, each day is in fact an emergency (somewhere). For we know not, never do we know, what the day, any day, can bring or will bring. Each day is an infinite set of possibilities. That's an emergency.

---

[6] Brian Andreas, "Story People: First Responder Print," accessed December 30, 2017, https://www.storypeople.com/2013/12/16/first-responder/.

It's one thing to philosophize about these things; it is quite another to be living and "becoming" through them, i.e., being shaped by them.

If you were or had been on the list I kept of people who loved Carolyn dearly, you would have received the following letter from me, her primary caregiver, who now had hosts of others carrying on the caregiving which can easily take over one's life:

To people who love Carolyn.

An update on Carolyn's and mine situation. The caring and love expressed by your calls, letters or cards went from you to me directly to Carolyn. Thank from both of us. We both needed that.

In her present circumstance, the majority of the time, she is in a peaceful tranquil state of mind and alert to her immediate surroundings. It is a far cry from how she was feeling and acting December, January and February prior to being hospitalized in a psychiatric unit to get stabilized on medications. The stabilization was a 17-day period of time which succeeded in that the meds began to cut down on the delusions which had increased in scope - from not recognizing me as her husband to not recognizing her own home. She also had great fears arising from a paranoia that people lived "upstairs and downstairs" (we have no up or down living quarters) and were out to hurt her. She could not understand how I who purported to want to be of help did not het rid of "those people." Some visual non-scary but strange hallucinations had begun to be a pattern. She became a flight risk.

From the psychiatric unit, she went to a skilled nursing facility (as some of you know) to wait for an opening at Arden Courts - the assisted living facility which specialized in memory care for Alzheimer's patients. Fortunately, she only had to stay at the crowded nursing unit for 10 days. On March 14th she was able to transfer to Arden Courts on Huebner where we expect and plan she will be permanently.

She is adjusting to the 3rd move in 30 days (from February 13th to March 14th) and, as I say, I am finding her in my daily visits, the majority of the time, to be tranquil and satisfied with the still fairly new surroundings. Been there a week today.

At present, all her quite nice furnishings are provided by Arden Courts. Little by little, I will be transferring furnishings from our home which I know she will love having - an orange leather chair, a grandmother's rocking chair, rugs we bought together, pictures from our walls - yeah! Lots of pictures - quilts passed on to her from grandmothers on both sides, etc., etc., etc.

The professionals and para pros at Arden Courts are sensitive to the various stages of impairment of their resident population. That takes their professionalism to a personal level of kindness and acceptance. Quite moving to see them bringing calmness and taking care.

8 to 9 different types of activities a day, 5 days are all geared - as you would guess - to provide the stimulus which promotes not only a comfortable environment but a pleasing and interesting one to be in. Nothing is pushed or forced but made inviting in respectful ways.

The tall wall surrounding the entire complex on the sides and rear allows the residents a place for walks in the outdoors should they choose that. Carolyn chose that the third day she was there. We had a hand-in-hand, joy-filled event. Simple things can mean so much. Like her knowing me as her husband now after 9 months of dealing with a stranger who became a friend. Before that walk she had not been outdoors to be outdoors in over a month.

So many things to be thankful and grateful for including Carolyn's foresight and shrewdness 17 years ago for having taken out that long-term care insurance making Arden Courts possible for us. Again, thanks for caring.

For those who plan to visit, please stay aware that the type and degree of her impairment allows no room for predicting how or when or why the mood can change.

You will notice that in that letter I alluded to eight or nine different (indoor) activities were provided five days a week at Arden Courts. Those varied from sing-a-longs of spiritual or popular songs to listening to small bands or choirs. All was quality entertainment which we family and friends were cordially invited to partake of with our loved one.

One of the reasons I began going to visit Carolyn in the mornings besides the afternoons and evenings was that I was told by staff of her hesitancy or outright refusal to go to the morning activities even though she was up and around. I interpreted this as a signal that Carolyn was depriving herself of needed stimulation so I took it upon myself to do the walking with her which I described earlier.

An added incentive for me to take on this frequency of visitations was that she was now recognizing me as the Edward she loved and had married. But this was only since the in-patient hospitalization preceding the 11 day stay at the nursing home and Arden Courts transfer. Prior to that, I have noted, Carolyn had gone for nine months without knowing me because of the syndrome, Capgras. I loved being known for who I was.

I just did not know how long that anti-psychotic medication would continue to hold the delusions at bay. By July 2014, four months after she arrived at Arden Courts and had successful results from that one medication, I dropped back my visitation from three times daily to two times daily every day of the week.

I would try to schedule my visits so that they did not coincide with some of the other regular visitors who most of which had a favorite day on which to go.

By July, too, Carolyn was a bit more inclined to accept my or a staffer's invitation to some of the activities in that big activity room.

A funny thing about that activity room from the beginning of her stay there: one time she and I were doing one of our indoor walks around the perimeter in the center of the four houses off of which stood the activity room. As we were walking in front of the then empty activity room, I motioned and asked Carolyn, "Do you want to go there?" She quickly jerked my arm away from that direction and spontaneously blurted out, "Don't go in there, they will start singing."

I laughed, and she let me know she was not laughing; enough said. We continued our walk.

In a letter which I sent to my list of Carolyn fans, I told them that Carolyn's ability to recognize me as her husband was absolutely huge on a number of levels. I wrote to them on April 11 of 2014:

This means many things on so many levels and one outstanding thing it means is that she can experience daily, when I go see her and as often as I go, that 'yes,' of course, her husband still loves her and is here for her - confusion not withstanding she knows (at some level) she is not alone. I thank you all, for both of us, for the prayers which reversed the seemingly impossible. Like the love song says! "No need to talk of tomorrow or forever." We will continue living the wonderful present, enjoying this renewal of life.

A particular superlative manifested itself at Arden Courts in the easy access I or her other caregivers had to the director and her administrative staff. They willingly shared feedback gleaned from all staff who dealt with Carolyn. This was the same with the nursing staff and the in-house psychiatrist. In April, for instance, the psychiatrist, an extremely competent and compassionate giver of care, shared with me that she surmised that Carolyn's rapid progression, in all probability, was due to what she believed was a vascular component to her Dementia. "With the vessels in the brain shrinking, the entire Alzheimer's process accelerates," she pointed out.

Her explanations enabled me to better understand the retrogenesis chart. And this enabled me to see the big picture and a context that explained why certain activities were beyond Carolyn's capacity.

CHAPTER FOURTEEN
THE CALIBRATION OF THE MOMENT

The painful calibration that, by April 2014, Carolyn was already at the moderate stage of Alzheimer's also told me that, though she was halfway down the scale, she was not yet at the end stages. Those stages were inevitable but she was not there yet. This provided more motivation for the frequency of good solid visits. It was like we had time to fill the energy tanks for the rougher road (journey? forest? paradox? Or plain reality!) ahead.

I shared copies of the retrogenesis chart with Carolyn's family and friends, informing them that the professionals at her memory care place whom I respected for their individual and cumulative years of experience considered the chart a fairly accurate measurement scale for the stages through which Alzheimer's patients go albeit at differing paces. "Here we have," I told them, "what we are looking at as we prepare for what's ahead." Later I found out that no amount of preparation really does it.

I also told them around this April that Carolyn continued exhibiting a peacefulness and a modicum of tranquility the majority of the time. I said in letters, "She gets annoyed at certain things but that does not last long and, best of all, she is no longer in a major fear of anything." Mostly, I reported to them, "She enjoys simple things. She responds to love, with love, not a bad place to be in."

I didn't tell them of one night and how she touched me deeply. I had done an evening ritual of foot and lower leg massage and my vibrational humming. Carolyn had fallen asleep. I had already helped her into her nightclothes and she lay there under the covers tucked in with love and affection. As I went to close her door, tiptoeing out, she opened her eyes and gazed at me. I said, "I love you, honey!" and she shot back, "I love you more." Wow! That was not an original expression but it was a clear communication - clear as a bell - when her communications all day had been undecipherable; it was a moment of momentous joy for me.

The ritual of helping her shed the day, by shedding the clothes she had worn that day, came about in quiet and a easy-flowing way. By evening, when I went to see her after their rather early supper at 4:30 p.m., Carolyn was pretty much ready to wind down. Occasionally we took a brief indoor or outside walk. Soon we were in her room and I was helping her don the evening with her nightclothes.

Since she was seeing me as her husband ever since the in-patient doctor was able to start her on the anti-psychotic medication, and her delusions as to who I was had subsided, she had no inhibitions with me slipping off her clothes - leaving her undergarments on - and helping her with her nightgown.

This practice automatically flowed like a seamless motion into one in which she raised her legs so that she was lying down and allowed me to sit at the foot of her bed in order to begin the foot and lower leg massage mentioned earlier. I started humming as soon as she lay back and closed the eyes of her body, allowing the relaxation and accompanying tranquility to simply be.

We both partook of the present quite effortlessly. Her look of serenity and surrender to the massage stimulated the release of my anxieties along with my bodily tension.

We weren't living together but it was amazing how close to one another we frequently were.

The closeness I speak of comprises the message I prepared and mailed to 37 relatives and friends both in town and in other cities.

The update enclosed deliberately excludes details which are too painful to recount.

I want to report what is missing that once was there and no longer is - but I would rather focus on what does exist that gives cause and reason to celebrate amidst the strangeness.

The strangeness is how we are experiencing two separate realities. Mine confuses her and her's I do not know how to penetrate.

And still we find a point of contact. We connect sufficiently for us both to experience that we are connecting and in a connection of love.

The love strengthens both our realities.

Now that is remarkable; and I call it prodigiously profound, because that is how I experience it.

Update on Carolyn as of August 4, 2014:

> *She now has little to no memory*
> *of hills and valleys to which we traveled.*
> *She now perceives landscapes*
> *unknown to me and unreportable by her;*
> *but we communicate love by touch*
> *and by the softness of soft but real kisses.*
> *Our mutual experiences are remarkably*
> *simple*
> *Yet prodigiously profound.*

I've learned to appreciate
Great beauty,

In the most minute of happenings
like the beauty in the smile of a woman
without guile and all the unmitigated
trust of a protected in the hands of a protector.
She's learned to seek me out
in what must be, to her, like unfamiliar forests
with unfamiliar roadways
and to find me in the midst of strangeness
coming out of nowhere leading
to who knows where.
I find her and she finds me and together
we travel to smaller hills and less deep valleys
and life goes on and
we live through good times
which are new ones.

And 'no' we do not speak of 'tomorrow' nor of
'forever'

I surprised myself, in re-reading some of my spasmodic journaling, that it took until May 2014 for me to surface in my consciousness that nothing in Carolyn's home belonged to her anymore. By then she had no memory of anything at home: not the pets (two cats which she had loved), not the jewelry which she had worn elegantly, and not the clothes of understated fashion which had graced her stylishly and now just hung motionless on hangers in her closets. She had no memory of the furnishings or the art we had enjoyed collecting together over the years.

My journaling faithfully reports amazement at my realization that Carolyn was still alive and here, yet I had already inherited everything. By prior arrangement she had left everything to me, just as I had willed everything to her were either of us to precede the other in death. Neither of us even remotely believed that one or the other would get to a mental state where home no longer felt or looked like the home we had furnished together. And here in the tenth home of our marriage we had lived for now 31 years.

As I have previously mentioned, in this tale of two lives and many more, Carolyn and I acted subconsciously as if I would naturally die first (barring all accidents) since I was nine years older. We knew an accident was possible for one or the other or both simultaneously; so, our wills were drawn up to cover all these possible eventualities.

To my total surprise, besides the one of awareness that I inherited everything, I never imagined how humble this would make me feel. I felt the weight of being undeserving because I sincerely believed - implicitly and explicitly - that she deserved this inheritance. My motive for savings throughout our marriage had been: "Yeah! That our old age be covered." But I saved, primarily, so Carolyn would not be stranded like many single women are without the means to have a comfortable assisted living preceding the end stages - whatever those might be - which life would send her or that which the Creator ordained!

I later realized that survivor's guilt was strongly impacting me. That's the guilt (blame) which arises when one feels one should have died instead of another. But I was experiencing this before Carolyn even died. I did not want to inherit our modest possessions if it meant the end of her life, especially while she was still alive. One more huge paradox.

I had no way, no force, no power to halt this concatenation of events.

The best I could do centered around the resolve, anew, to be the best caregiver I could be in order to make the trainload of events Carolyn was enduring to be as great as I could make them.

In the evenings at home where I retreated alone every night after the last visit of the day, I seriously gave thought to what I wanted to consciously mean by "…great as I could make them (her events)." I wanted to rise above the cliché which that could become; so, I carefully examined whether I wanted "great" to be: fun? happy? comfortable? peaceful? loving?

I concluded that, to be truly loving, nurturing, and affectionate, everything else would fall into place. I was simply using women like Carolyn as my role model.

In those alone nights I also pondered what had been part of my cognitive restructuring intervention with patients in my 31 years as a psychotherapist, especially with those who had caregiver roles. With them I always covered the ground embedded in the Latin: "*Nemo dat, quam non habet,*" for "no one gives what one does not have."

In that cognitive restructuring intervention, I helped my patients look for what they needed to attend to in order for their lives to continue growing in their various facets, in spite of the giant vortex trying to swallow them up. We would explore what could be done in their immediate life (the one going with care-taking) to maintain physical, mental, and emotional health. We also explored their social and spiritual health - however it was that they viewed the life of their spirit.

I proceeded to attend to staying healthy in all these facets of my life. I did this partially by teaching myself what others had been taught by me.

The many people who showed great love and attentiveness to Carolyn and to me also reminded me frequently to take care of myself. Their teaching succeeded.

It seems so obvious that one cannot impart peacefulness if one does not cultivate it, but nothing could be less peaceful than to have one's life subsumed by the needs of one desperately needing to be taken care of all of the time! Many a mother's total life has been swallowed up by the needs of a disabled child or a brew of "normal" children.

Dementia patients go to that stage of infancy where you and I were when we could neither say please nor thank you. We didn't because we couldn't.

It takes mountains of effort for the caretakers of Dementia patients to carve out time in the 24-hour-day to go, not to, as someone pointed out, where one says: "me first!" but to where one says: "me too!"

Luckily, fortunately, blessedly, I had sufficient reminders from my own past and from the present relatives, friends, and professionals around me to take care of myself. So, I did and I was able to be one of many sources for calming energy to Carolyn. I was able to provide peaceful atmosphere alongside a host of others.

Had I not done the exercises to keep the body, mind, and spirit well-nourished and strong, things like survivor's guilt could have taken me to dark and dangerous places.

CHAPTER FIFTEEN
THE UNDERBELLY OF THE MOMENT

It turned out that, as of July 2014, I would start seeing Carolyn twice a day instead of three times. She had started showing less resistance to attending the many morning indoor activities provided by Arden Courts. It seemed healthier for her to do more socializing with the larger group. This also meant one less walk per day for us, but the replacement of indoor interrelationship activity seemed like a balanced trade off.

The significant changes in August 2014 are reflected in my journaling account of August 12, 2014:

The eerie feeling is back, like the feelings one gets when you can almost feel the whisper of the axe which is about to fall and chop off a major chunk from life as we know it. More and more signs of decline in Carolyn's condition tell less and less of what she can give to us anymore. She is becoming more impersonal, because she must feel less personal due perhaps 'cause she doesn't know what to feel nor, maybe how to feel.'

Three days ago, as we walked down one hallway she asked me - very personally, by the way - "Do you think I'm losing my mind?" My immediate response was non-alarmed sounding: "I don't believe so!" Then, I asked, "Why do you think that?" She replied that it just felt that way when she did not understand, and then could not say what she did not understand.

That conversation ended as abruptly as it had started. I stayed silently startled. She is more and more fatigued, frequently, it seems like (sic). It takes a couple of breaths with her eyes closed and she is asleep. She responds to the feet massage instantly, like I say, a couple of breaths and she is on her way to being out; she registers joy or delight over a familiar face, but cannot sustain it longer than an instant in time. She shows aimlessness more frequently and for longer periods of time. All new behaviors. On the other hand, she seems to interact more with staffers (the CNA's who watch over them). They all show a very positive regard for her and they let her know they welcome the attention she favors them with. They certainty favor her with much fond, genuine, sincere attention.

I am finding good energy boosts in the weekly meditation group I joined now 5 weeks ago and the every-other-day gym exercise of an hour of upper and lower body work-out. I am attempting to read heavy stuff like sutras by Ashtavakra and lighter stuff like Bless Me Ultima *and* Time *and* Smithsonian *magazines to form a balance. Just to stay rounded.*

By August 13, 2014, Carolyn had been gone from our home for five whole months, and I was not feeling a pressing need to move from where we had been living. When I had been anticipating the eventuality that I would need to place Carolyn in an environment where three shifts of professional caretakers would have to watch her, I naturally assumed that I would have to consider next where I would go live. I knew I had options, such as a small apartment or a retirement community for independent living. In either of those cases, I could sell our home or consider renting it out.

Several friends volunteered to help me move as soon as I chose my next home.

It was not long after I placed Carolyn at Arden Courts that I made the decision not to decide for at least eight months to year; certainly not before.

I eased into the living alone and was determined to maintain the home as cleanly and tidily as Carolyn always had. I learned to thoroughly enjoy living in the whole house.

My major adjustment which went the least gracefully was "what to eat?" or "where to eat?" She and I had begun the buying of pre-prepared frozen microwaveable meals as described earlier. Somehow, the fact that I now needed to adjust to eating alone made the whole pattern of eating a difficult one to establish. Some close friends volunteered to teach me to cook. One bought me The Four Ingredients Cook Book which is like the "how to" for dummies in the cooking department. I never did learn. Never did try.

I had always thoroughly loved the home we had put together and how we had done it. It all grew on me in a renewed sort of way. My attachment to everything we owned became an even more prized possession. Strangely, too, grew the desire to share many of the beautiful possessions which decorated all the rooms of our two-bedroom home.

There lingered in my subconsciousness the thought that, in the very near future, I would be moving out. So, after five months of living on my own, I had dispossessed myself of quite a few items.

To various family members I gave four hallway runners and other throw rugs from various rooms. I gave away our dining room table and eight dining room chairs in order to clear that room for something which Carolyn had long-time-ago thought of doing: to make that space an office.

A favorite collection of mine was a set of seven decanters - mostly cut glass - passed on to me personally by Carolyn's mom. I gave these to seven different households. Some beautiful pottery (from Carolyn's kitchen) went to some of her friends in her name.

More pottery which had been precious to us also found new homes. Her antique bedspreads went to new bedrooms in homes of nieces, as I knew Carolyn would have directed.

Some of our possessions found their way to Carolyn's room at Arden Courts so that its entire furnishing, save for a bed and one immovable closet, consisted of possessions from our home.

Even with all that gone from the house, nothing seemed to be missing, because there was plenty more to replace all those giveaways.

Fortunately, I had taken time to photograph all the art and wall hangings in our house and had made 4 x 6 prints. Very carefully, like one cuts paper dolls, I cut out the images of these works of art and composed what turned out to be much more than a scrapbook. It is a book about art which, even if I say so myself, is a work of art by itself. It is a one of a kind; a *"sui generis"* work of art.

Some of the energy from one pronounced creative streak channeled me into rearranging some of the art pieces on all our walls. The kitchen was the least affected by my drive to reposition and collocate differently.

I had loved Carolyn's choice of what went where but the walls clamored for changes.

Much went into dedicating a considerable amount of new stuff in the guest bedroom so that it reflected a significant place for memorabilia about Carolyn. I love the way it's turned out...with many more pictures of her which tell various stories about her.

One did not have to go too deeply into my subconsciousness to see that I was reshaping my environment according to me.

My evenings alone turned into some TV watching, once I returned from the evening rituals with Carolyn and whatever or wherever I ate. I also spent time photographing, cutting out art pieces from the photos I had taken, and pasting in a large book with spiral binding. Doing soft pastel (chalk) works of art became another evening occupation.

The soft pastels and, later, watercolor works eventually made up a gallery out of two garage walls.

All of these activities, coupled with what I packed up and gave away, served to help me face the newness and strangeness which life was presenting me as Carolyn made her way to the retrogenesis endemic to Alzheimer's' disease.

"Facing the newness and strangeness" was an ongoing process. Some of it flowed smoothly; some, not so accommodating as all that.

The resources for this journey for both Carolyn and myself were innumerable and they stood in such relief that only an obtuse fool would have failed to appreciate their value. As you would guess, the most valuable resources were people.

Playing our favorite CD's when I engaged in all those activities other than TV watching was a tremendous source of beautiful recollection. It also provided a backdrop for the creation of new memorable memories, whether of newly experienced vulnerabilities or the saving of this or that new awareness of the love which still flowed between our ever-changing lives.

My readings, my writings, and particularly the many human interactions with relatives and friends who did not leave us out of their social, physical, and spiritual sight, all contributed to an acceptance of Carolyn exactly as the day presented her to us and an enjoyment in the doing and being for her.

This acceptance of her exactly as she was on the given day precluded much sorrow and pain for what she was no more. Her growing distance from our reality meant she went further into her reality which we knew nothing about except that it was as real to her as ours is to us. Up until this time Carolyn still knew herself in her reality. What dramatically appeared now in August 2014 did not indicate that she knew herself even in the reality she was experiencing. In the past, she could also tell us when she felt tired. Now fatigue appeared and she merely succumbed without a word about it.

As I mentioned earlier, she seemed without aim. Aimlessness and lack of acknowledgment of things and events in our reality was becoming more pronounced.

For the next four months, August through December, Carolyn did continue responding to the touch of the foot and lower leg massage and to the vibrations of the accompanying humming.

She continued inviting that experience with ready acquiescence and mild but real pleasure, closing the eyes and obviously releasing physical tension and slowly breathing though a relaxing experience which would morph into what resembled a centeredness and peacefulness of spirit and culminate in a deep sleep.

Carolyn would awaken in 10 to 15 minutes, utter one or two sentences, re-close the eyes, and resume her deep sleep. 10 or 15 minutes later this pattern reappeared. It usually did not happen more than twice or three times, and then she was out for the night. I had no way of knowing how many times she re-awakened after I left. Staff usually reported to me next afternoon how soundly she had slept.

I want to insert a section of my journaling of August 25, 2014, to give the reader an idea of the types of welcomed non-planned, non-scripted events which gave me unusual, out of the ordinary resources for coping in order to keep living my life (the one I needed to maintain). While I deeply felt I devoted two-thirds of my life to my role as caregiver, I was experiencing Carolyn less and less devoted to a life of us together.

Two-thirds of my life would mathematically be 16 hours of my day. I do not want to deceive and declare that I was giving 16 hours a day to attending to Carolyn. I do want to say that it felt like that was what I was doing, even when she was already in a place where she was watched day and night. That was an enormous relief. But the load still felt enormous.

Hard to believe XMAS is upon us in 4 months only. Somebody whose mother has died of Alzheimer's told me the other day: "part of what you are going through is that everybody's life keeps going on around you and yours isn't… because you are care-taking" and that is so true. I was thinking that because I am conscious to stay in touch with other aspects of life besides the tragic one going on with Carolyn's decline (in Dementia) and going deeper and deeper into retrogenesis, I am, in fact, going on with my life- to some extent. I am, but, I am not, in a sense, living apart from Carolyn.

A full 2/3 of my day life seems wrapped around care for her, in spite of the fact that she has now been in a facility for 6 months where they daily take care, as best they can, of every need. I say, "as best they can" because I have gone at times and it was a good thing I went when I did because none of the custodians were there to attend to an immediate need. I took care of the need she had. I did not fault anyone if they could not bi-locate and serve more than two patients at a time. 3 separate times - all bathroom issues - I was there, thankfully, to go take care of an emergent need."

(What this all referred to was the fact that Carolyn had been slipping into urinary incontinence. This had just begun to happen occasionally and it was not known to all her care-takers yet).

How many other times have there been emergent needs and neither I nor a staff person was there to extricate her from the problem at hand?? No one knows. The place she is in, is wonderful, but like all else in life, it is not perfect, so, no, I am not lodging a complaint.

...I am doing things which she cannot participate in, which fulfill some of my social, spiritual, emotional, intellectual, and physical needs (not sure if I am attending to the whole Maslow hierarchy of needs). I do lunches, dinners... go to weekly group meditation, do a private meditation daily... go to the gym every other day (usually)... laundry... grocery shopping... artwork... some writing, not as much as a writer does when one is faithful to that profession... want to be engaged in writing as if it were my profession... need to improve on this, correspondence, (long hand, old school) with a number of wonderful friends... periodically do mail outs of updates to 20 or 40 people in Carolyn's and my life.

On an inspiration, I awoke from a brief morning nap and took myself to Houston and Flores streets downtown where I parked free cause it was Sunday. I walked 2 or 3 blocks to the San Fernando Cathedral. The inspired thought had been to go visit that place designated as sacred by Catholics where throngs gather to synergistically join in petitioning the Ultimate Reality whom they refer to as G-O-D in the form of

Jesus of Nazareth, his Father God the Father and a Holy Spirit whom they believe emanates as the love between the father and the Son (whom they believe became incarnate and was called the Christ, Jesus). 3 separate persons sharing one divine nature.

I know all of this because I too was once a proponent of these beliefs.

The last time I had been in that beautifully restored and renovated sacred place was with Carolyn and her dad. We had taken him to see, one Sunday morning, how that holy place had been redone. That has to have been 12 years ago. My strong and compelling desire as I awoke had been "go visit the cathedral and maybe the Mercado. Get a good walk in, take yourself to be among people - many of whom will be there because it is Sunday, and Sundays are for congregating to pray together, go, go and see. Go and observe. Observe once more but with renewed interest, or perhaps with a renewed ability to observe.

So, I went and I observed and the current took me to a Sunday 12 noon Mass.

I had had no intention of going to a mass. I was in shorts; like the ones tourists wear... there were very few people milling in front of the church; some were sitting in shaded areas... some ambulating, like me, around the 3 or 4 multi-water fountains spurting up from ground level, all simple and picturesque.

Walked into the church and found it maybe half full of people. It was 25 minutes' till noon. I had not seen the interior in years, and, sure enough! it gave me a semi-deep sigh and semi-breathless feeling. It was as wondrously beautiful as I thought I had remembered it.

The reredos (background to an altar) is spectacular in its gold reflection. The nave takes your perception in and you feel pulled into a wonderful feeling. The center altar - now facing the people - is a huge square table (like butcher tables are) of a solid-looking piece - huge beautiful piece - of marble or precious stone. Giant candle sticks of brass, 8 or 10 of them border the outer edges from the floor on up.

The high wooden pulpit, the steps leading up to the altar, the red candle burning in a hanging red candle holder, the cleanly arranged flower bases, the fabrics, the stone of the walls reaching up to where incense rises, stained glass windows, all deep in the nave, towards the front of this house of prayer, all come together to form a tableau of simplicity with the power of "just there" to behold.

Along the side walls of the Cathedral are these immense sculptures of clusters of figures - 14 in all - the stations of the cross, of course. One finds 14 such stations in all Catholic churches though few are as magnificent a work of art as these are. All tastefully sculpted and collocated masterfully.

Most of the seating naturally faces the front but now there appear seats towards the front of the altar which face towards the altar from its sides, thus those seats face each other from the left side of the church to be right side and vice versa. There also includes seating between the altar now used and the one at the back wall which used to be used. That back wall facing the congregation contains the reredos which was shipped to Mexico City and back and returned in all its ornamentation and ornamentalism.

As I allowed myself the vision of my consciousness to take in all of this interior to my inner self, I felt like I could increasingly appreciate why this place is designated sacred ground, house of G-O-D.

In 25 minutes from my arrival the entire church became packed with serious looking but not somber people. Kind countenances.

At 12 noon sharp, a procession emerged from the front entrance to the altar: acolytes in cassocks and surplices with candles in tow: one with a crucifix mounted on a high brass pole; one with a thurible (container for charcoal) burning with incense; one with an oversized book followed by a sub deacon, a deacon and the main celebrant the one with a chasuble - two-sided garment falling in front and back of the celebrant.

They all followed their specified roles while pontificating a ritualized high mass, complete with lay readers and lay people distributing communion, all solemn, very moving. All "just there" for the experience. I soon forgot I was wearing the shorts which I had thought were going to persuade me to leave before I got caught up in the mood furthered by a powerful choir.

CHAPTER SIXTEEN
THE "LONG GOOD-BYE" OF THE MOMENT

Visits from out-of-town relatives and friends added great variety, constituting yet another unscripted resource to draw upon. Carolyn had long ago stopped communicating about our reality, but these people came anyway because they wanted to express their love and concern for her and for us the caretakers. Fortunately, there occurred many out of town visits, especially from her niece Eileen from Montgomery.

That niece has known of the solicitous care Carolyn extended towards her mom's five sisters in the Dallas area. Carolyn had always loved those aunts and their husbands dearly. She took a special interest in their geriatric years by going to Dallas frequently to help them with financial or health affairs.

Eileen knew this about her aunt Carolyn and modeled herself after her by being the faithful niece who came frequently to San Antonio to see and care for both of us. She was a great comfort to me as well. Her sister Emily, who also displayed much love for her Aunt Carolyn, resided in Finland with her two daughters and husband. That geographic distance precluded coming frequently.

Late August of 2014 saw the unfolding of another serious omen of decline besides the beginnings of urinary incontinence. This was Carolyn doing what we had observed others of advanced Dementia doing. She had begun going into open doors of empty rooms and falling asleep - fully clothed - on top of someone else's bed in early afternoon. Fortunately, she didn't close the door behind her so I would find her, gently awaken her so as to not startle her, and guide her to her own bed if she wanted to continue her nap.

On occasion, Carolyn did close the door behind her. In this case I let staff find her in order that I might have an afternoon visit with her. I did not take it upon myself to open closed doors.

When escorted to her own room, Carolyn always followed meekly and compliantly without saying a word and apparently was totally oblivious to the simple act of infringing on someone else's space.

Once or twice I found her sitting on the edge of someone's bed gazing at the floor; she was not in a daze as much as gazing with no thought process going on. This paucity of thought is a condition appearing in patients who experience fewer and fewer thoughts in their waking state and for prolonged periods of time.

The third pattern to arise was her carrying some of her picture frames from her room and leaving them in other places like the dining room, kitchen, someone else's room, the TV room etc. She also dismantled all stands on those picture frames.

Before this August ended with the sting of these latter developments portentous of more radical changes in Carolyn's personality, I was fortunate to participate in two totally different group experiences. These separate experiences contributed enormously to reshaping my enthusiasm for life and my passion for living it fully. They also gave me the enlightening inspiration to stay awake (aware, centered, mindful) to life as it comes inexorably upon us daily (whether we are ready or not).

One group consisted of fellow caregivers whom I had met early in the year when Arden Courts treated us all with the eight-week "Stress-Busting Program for Caregivers." I have also stated why that was such a meaningful living experience.

An extension of that experience was that a group of eight or nine of us had derived so much from the experiential component that we chose to continue meeting once the formal program ended. We were meeting almost monthly at a local restaurant to catch up on how our loved ones were doing and how we were coping. Everyone's loved one was in varying stages of Dementia. For some time, we had all felt that of all our acquaintances, perhaps it was the people in this group who better grasped the significance of our vulnerabilities. We met together because we liked each other and we felt free to talk with one another. In my journal, after our August meeting, I had noted how that gathering made me strongly realize how far from being alone I really was. I had known that, but somehow the realization of it was forcefully made. Hence my attribution to those people for renewed enthusiasm, passion, and inspiration.

The second powerful group experience occurred at a place where, just two months prior, I had enrolled to be trained to be a volunteer for a program to open later that December.

The program to be was a contemplative home for death and dying. In August there was an extensive and intensive workshop for several of us who hoped to be ready as volunteers when the doors were projected to be opened just before Christmas.

The program exposed us to the physical signs of dying and the spiritual signs of impending death. There we contemplated the mystery of death and the mystery of life.

The one-day exposure to the tip of the iceberg of death and dying profoundly moved and enriched us. The content of it all could not have come at a better time for me. It did indeed imbue me with enthusiasm, passion, and inspiration. I felt, also, the nascent feelings for a group of men and women who were destined to become, for me, like family.

Somewhere in my psyche roamed around the sentiments of the value I was losing in Carolyn's departure from our reality and my life. Somewhere in there, too, was enfolded the need to add new value, preferably in the form of human relationships as those of a family. The reality of her slipping away and bringing about her "long good-bye" prompted me on September 3, 2014, to write the following to relatives and friends in and out of town.

I am strongly moved (at times) to play her music (music she's liked). So that it fills every room in this whole house. Just like that self-same music has - over the years - filled my whole soul.

And when I do just that, by finding a favorite (past) album of her's and turn up the volume to 'fill this house entirely,' my whole soul sways with the vibrating windows and a lampshade or two, and I wonder when the first time was that she heard this one for the last time.

She's begun to do scores of every day doings 'for the last time' and doing that many more times. Just saying.

Like she's cooked for the last time and driven her car - any car - for the last time. And even eye-lined her eyes with eye-liner for the last time.

She no longer goes to movies, nor does she ask for pets, nor home, nor clothing once dear to her taste.

She's read her last novel, I'm sure, and now, no button sews, does not read mags and asks not: How the news goes.

She's in retrogenesis like we all, someday, will be and that's simply when we are gently let down to where we were when we were being raised up (i.e. the human in Dementia returning to infancy). When we were being raised up, we were, as it were, like rosebuds growing to where we'd bloom.

After our bloom, comes a descent to where flowers originate, that is, to basic elements, to earth.

Many a garden has bloomed from just such basic elements. (To use Mother Nature's seasons, for example). Just saying."

You can see that, amidst the pain of all she can no longer do and the inevitability of returning to the dust from which we came, I'm reminding myself and those who grieve for Carolyn in "the long good-bye," that that transformation awaits her and us.

Specifically, what triggered the writing of September 3, 2014, was an incident wherein Carolyn suddenly appeared in the breakfast room looking like either a raccoon or like someone who just received two black eyes in a physical fight, and this before visitors who were there to see her for lunch! She had just lost her sense of how to apply mascara to her eyes - nothing more and nothing less - but the result was quite a spectacle. I do know that one visitor was mortified when she reported to me that Carolyn had gotten two black eyes in some painful incident. Why the CNA's on duty had not cleaned her face before I requested that they do so, I never inquired. It may have been funny or hilarious to some; to me it was one more thing she could no longer do and that was hurtful to the quick. That same afternoon I removed all makeup and brushes and nail polish and took it home - just thinking for the first time of what Carolyn had now done for her last time.

For some quirky reason it would take a long time before I could let go of those two images of Carolyn from my memory. What continued popping up in my mind's eye was a stark scene of someone else's room there at Arden Courts. In this neatly made up, very home-like atmosphere (just like Carolyn's was), Carolyn was fully clothed and lying there in a semi-fetal position, sound asleep and not aware when awakened why anyone would find it strange for her to be asleep in the middle of the day. The scene carried no danger whatsoever, it was just the announcement that Carolyn had made one more leap away from our consciousness. Another giant leap.

The other scene which also frequently popped out as if it, too, had an important message to convey, was Carolyn standing there with two huge black circles surrounding each of her eyes and, she, totally oblivious to how bizarre that look was outside of a scary movie.

Both scenes, for me, represented a painful reality which was fraught with helplessness for a little girl; one unaware of her vulnerability and of the fact that all the people surrounding her were to be her protectors.

To this day both recollections evoke a silent humming of that old popular song with these lyrics: "and when I cry, my eyes are dry the tears are in my heart." [7]

By the time all this transpired I had begun warning out of town visitors that their plan for a visit might not be a visit at all.

The following is a verbatim letter to one of Carolyn's dearest cousins and it pretty well spells out what I wrote to others who were planning to make a final trip:

Dear Nancy Marie,

---

[7] Perry Como with Lloyd Shafer and His Orchestra, "Laughing on the Outside (Crying on the Inside)," *"Live" at the Supper Club 1946*, Sounds of Yesteryear, CD.

If you still want to come to see Carolyn after you read what I'm about to risk saying, by all means please know you are abundantly welcome to come and stay at our home. We have one guest bedroom and plenty of couch space in the living room - you get the Bedroom!

Carolyn can no longer give what and "how" she could before her Alzheimer's got to this stage. You already know that. Know, too, she cannot have a conversation.

She cannot answer questions in a manner that gives a meaning to what's asked.

She asks questions which are undecipherable. She can show a genuine glee when she first sees someone from her past whom she vaguely recognizes but she cannot sustain the glee for more than a second or two. Almost immediately she's now "talking" to that person with words which do not make sense.

The words do not make sense either cause the listener has no idea who or what they are referring to or the words are jumbled up to where subjects and predicate are confused or the words she chooses have no meaning as they are used or all of the above at once.

She's clearly experiencing something in a reality different from the one the listener is in and, as I say, the language she uses is not in a form we can grasp.

This means visitors from out of town can come visit with her and have no idea what or whom she is perceiving just like me who sees her daily. Most of the time I believe she knows it was Ed her husband who came and visited her.

She has frequently had a woman friend come see her and I know it cause I saw the name in the sign-in-sign out ledger and I ask her whether her friend was there to see her and 90% of the time she says "no" or she "didn't find her" or she (Carolyn) "wasn't there" or she "doesn't remember." I believe those visits have a value in that they keep her sense of "I am considered a special friend" alive. That sense may not have much staying power but when reinforced by another visit by someone else, cumulatively taken, all the visits keep her sense of who she is alive if only in her reality if not ours. In her reality, she knows who she is. Most of the time, even this has begun to slip away.

I hope this makes some sense, I am trying to describe what's obviously to me, an extremely complex... "complexity" (for lack of another word).

I know that a Dallas to San Antonio trip means 4 to 5 hours one way and I know that visits with Carolyn for longer than say 20 minutes can become very arduous - not for lack of love - but for lack of knowing what to say next and how to handle this or that intonation of her voice so she can feel there's a connection there. When she feels there's no connection, she literally moves on. She steps away and starts heading somewhere else. That's not the old Carolyn.

Its disconcerting to me who is learning daily to not be surprised; it's the stuff that's brought some of her visitors to tears when she's not looking. I am trying to say it's God-awful painful.

There are a number of salvific things about all this and one is, as I say, in her reality she has an identity, in our reality she is lost like in that unfamiliar forest I once alluded to.

Also, since she's not in touch with our reality, the things of this world are of no concern and therefore no worry to her. She is relatively stress-free compared to us who worry about the hairs on our head and who frequently forget what we were told about the "lilies in the field who neither spin not do they sew" etc. etc. etc.

She does continue to eat well and heartedly I am told repeatedly.

She goes to sleep in what she now considers her space her bed, with a relaxation of the feet by, me, her faithful companion whom more often than not, she now sees as her husband and the husband she loves (sometimes when I tell her I love her, she shoots back "I love you more.") so the relaxed mood is accompanied by a calm and peaceful mood when she traipses off to sleep every night.

The people there have grown to like her a lot so I know the care she receives even when we, the family, aren't looking is genuine.

Give me a call.
Ciao, con mucho cariño (Bye and with much caring)
                                    Ed

Hopefully, that letter indicates how much I told out-of-towners. You can see how much more was going on which others could not possibly imagine unless they, too, had been a care taker of one with Alzheimer's.

CHAPTER SEVENTEEN
THE HEAVINESS OF THE MOMENT

The holidays had begun with the coming and passing of Thanksgiving. Few of the residents at Arden Courts could appreciate to any great depth what had been prepared for Thanksgiving dinner and what was being prepared for Christmas.

We the relatives and friends of the patients reacted with joy and laughter, literally, to what staff did and was doing for the holidays. The purpose of creating a mood was accomplished and everyone benefitted either way directly or at least indirectly.

Family and friends were motivated to do our own decorating in the room of our beloved.

The following account specifies what I wrote and told Carolyn's fans about what I had done to bring the Christmas spirit to her immediate surroundings:

December 5, 2014

I have introduced some Christmas decorations to Carolyn's home away from home (the one I am in, is still hers).

The top shelf above her bed in her apartment has seen a replacement of childhood toys (which had been saved for her by one of her aunts) with one angel on each end (girl angels at that) one ceramic Santa next to each of the angels, then one brass and bronze deer (looking as if mesmerized not by head lights, but by an invisible giant star illuminating the silent night and the noisy day). Next to the brass/bronze ones are smaller, but no less imposing, chrome deer - and oh! The bronze ones hold a purple- as in royal- candle each. Then, in the very center of the shelf I placed a wooden horse- a tad bigger than the four deer as in real life - red and with a green bridle and it rocks like horsies of kids of all ages do, and suspended from the rocking horse is a rocking red-red-and-glittery Christmas stocking with the name, Carolyn, emblazoned upon it - that came from her mama, Sara Sherblom of Helotes, Texas decades ago- and we've hung it at our fire place ever since.

Attached to the XMAS stocking but unseen by the un-trained eye is a smaller XMAS stocking made by Cookie out of material from one of K.A.'s neck ties. Carolyn loved that memento of her cherished brother.

On her English writing table facing her bed I have placed a silver shiny angel whose gender cannot be determined from sight alone. This one is much bigger than the two on the shelf. She had bought this one at the Morningside gift shop where she volunteered, so that ornamentation brings her a special energy from Morningside for being the special place it has been in her life.

On her dresser at the deeper part of her room, stands a majestic tree made of iron, brown iron bars holding hearts, stars, bird-shapes, crosses, half-moons, etc. all hanging off the iron bars.

It stands maybe 30 inches high and at its widest extension measures maybe 24 or so inches.

The little hanging thingies are iron plate: little hearts and clover leafs and flowers and what looks like fruit which could be pears.

On the very top of this unusually beautiful sculpture sits, what I call, a partridge on a pear tree. Carolyn had bought that also at the gift shop where she volunteered. That was her last purchase there - 3 years' ages? Ago?

The wreath we used on our front door fashioned with reindeer bells (bells which go around the neck of Christmas deer) on wire and a flowing array of make-believe-greenery-and-berries and ribbons (red red, of course) takes the place of the work of art Sue Ellen had created for her in the form of a wreath with secret pouches and pull-out pins and fiesta colors which has graced her door at Arden Courts since fiesta San Antonio.

The Sue Ellen wreath is safely ensconced in the bottom drawer of her dresser with the childhood toys, all in hibernation 'till the merriment of XMAS blows over for another type of "let's celebrate."

So, there you have it evidence of "as the world turns."

I wish that I could report that she loved it all; she registered no emotion one way or another to the decorations which many complimented her on.

Although a decrement had set in to Carolyn's ability to emote and to respond to emotions, I had definitely felt a pronounced increment to the amount and quality of social contact as a result of mailing out updates on our road to Alzheimer's.

The amount and content of cards, letters, and phone calls was very fulfilling. To have received an average of 19 to 20 responses -

all positive and full of genuine love - out of every 33 to 35 mail outs like the one of December 5, 2014 was nothing short of gratifying.

Not near 100% response rate but the positive content of responders had been absolutely wonderful.

In my mail outs, I charted phenomena which I witnessed going on during the unfolding of the enfolded journey in Alzheimer's as manifested by Carolyn's behaviors and experienced by those of us up-close to the daily unfurling. I had once read of a concept in a Japanese philosophy referred to as *Shibumi*. "It is a statement so correct that it does not have to be bold, so poignant it does not have to be pretty, so true it does not have to be real."[8]

In my mail outs, I intended to write true statements and poignant ones about what we encountered in this path to retrogenesis as it unfolded in our lives. We followed the path taking Carolyn. She did not choose the path; the path had chosen her.

Sometime between August and September, a poignant event almost took me to a depressed state. By that time Carolyn's psychiatrist advised me to put Carolyn permanently on Depends (the undergarment worn by people who have reached urinary incontinence). I had been preparing for this eventuality so, of course, I could readily agree with her as soon as she told me. What happened next blew me away.

A day or two after this talk with the doctor, I was standing between the kitchen and the dining room of the green house talking with the CNA who had come on duty at 6:00 a.m. I was enjoying a chat with this CNA whom Carolyn showed great attachment to by the way she often tried to be her kitchen helper, when up came another CNA who also worked on the unit. This CNA handed me a large clear plastic zip-lock bag containing four neatly-folded pairs of

---

[8] Trevanian, *Shibumi*, (Outlet: 1979), 77.

Carolyn's underwear. The woman said, as she handed me the bag, "You know, she no longer needs her panties."

That simple non-ceremonious act struck a nerve - the one we feel at the center of our gut-when we intuitively perceive that a finality has arrived and "something" will be no more.

Momentarily, my world's motion came to a dead halt.

I had understood the psychiatrist's pronouncement about Depends. The finality behind the reality had not hit me like it did when the clear plastic bag appeared like the flag handed to the grieving family of a service person being buried.

The chill over me, in that agonizing instant, took the form of "I am burying Carolyn." To be perfectly frank, I did not know at that time why I had the chill. It took several days of reliving that moment and discussing it with precious few before I could go back and semi-identify what my subconsciousness was carrying - equating plastic bag with ritual of a burial. The memory remains firmly implanted in my emotional make up.

Here it was September of 2014 and Capgras had not appeared for eight wonderful months. Other losses were taking place: losses of abilities, of skills, and of interest in many areas of life. Just recently it appeared as if she lost the sense of herself as a person. And now on September 9, 2014, I recorded in my journal that in that week it appeared as if Edward, the man she recognized as her husband, had for those eight months disappeared from her experience.

That realization brought the hurt all over again.

This time the disappearance was not marked by an awareness or by a manifestation of an awareness by Carolyn. I just perceived being seen as a familiar face but not as a husband. She simply accepted the new "given" as just that - a "given" like the given that now somebody helped her change clothes at night and someone else dressed her in the morning. And if no one changed her at night, why, she just slept in her day's clothes and if no one dressed her in the morning she stayed in nightclothes until someone did. So it seemed that if her husband no longer came, she simply accepted the one who did come. I had stated earlier in Carolyn's descent along the seven stages of retrogenesis that not only did she not know how to tie her shoe laces, or make the bed, or drive her car but that she arrived at a point where she did not know that at one time she did know how to do all those things. That was my perception of Capgras now in this September since she had come to Arden Courts; Carolyn did not seem to know that there was once an Edward, the husband. This was not easy to stomach.

I had been actively practicing acceptance of Carolyn as she was, choosing to not focus on what we had had together for 46 years and who she had been in those 46 years. It suddenly became even more of a challenge to accept her as one who could not know that she was once my wife.

The "letting go" that this reality presented became one of the toughest to do.

Various events changed my relationships with various relatives because of new behaviors of theirs and how those behaviors impacted negatively the rest of the family, but they paled in comparison to the impact which Carolyn's change was now having on me.

Fortunately, the many resources which I have enumerated served to bring me the healing my wounded-ness needed, the strength to offset the tiredness and fears, the hope to keep from feeling enfolded by helplessness, some joy to prevent depression, and my success over things within my purview of control. This latter resource I needed, especially, to ward off "failure."

It took some time for my awareness to see this new development as, very probably, a natural consequence of Carolyn's losing her sense of self. That, of course, was due to the mind shutting down just as we had been witnessing the body shutting down.

It goes without saying that, had it not been for meditation on a daily basis, I would not have been able to pull all the resources together to accept and not despair, or go into anger, or find fault with life for what all of us encounter in this facet of life.

My journal abounds with my experiences of meditation and how that became the resource for having access to all the other resources.

Specifics which meditation kept me in touch with included a consciously developed list of "things I do not need to do":

- *I do not need to take myself too seriously*
- *I do not need to lose whatever degree of centeredness I have arrived upon*
- *I do not need to pretend that I have arrived*
- *I do not need to be a cynic*
- *I do not need to pretend that I need no one*
- *I do not need to act as if I can't*
- *I do not need to ignore the presence of energy just because it is as invisible as gravity*
- *I do not need to forget that, as of today, there are an infinite set of possibilities, an equal train of probabilities, and a commensurate number of certainties; and that, as a human, I too am an infinite set of possibilities*
- *I do not need to forget we all have a watchful Creator*
- *I do not need to forget the life principle that there is purpose to everything that happens and there is also purpose and meaning to everything I do; positive or negative depending on my focus*
- *I do not need to ignore music nor others*

- *I do not need to chide myself or give up because I lose focus or mindfulness; just need to return to it*
- *I do not need to stand still, but improve what is in my power*
- *I do not need to "not grow"*
- *I do not need to ignore "just being" and observing and growing with the experience*

These themes suggested to me what to cultivate in meditative mood instead of what to fall into. My list of "I do not need" identifies as my primary list of vulnerabilities - the roads I need not travel and paths I wanted to keep avoiding.

CHAPTER EIGHTEEN
THE LIGHT AND SHADOW OF THE MOMENT

By December 2014 Carolyn had descended to the sixth of seven stages of the retrogenesis ladder. She had journeyed in and out and in and out of Capgras for a total of two years and seven months. By this time, in her many cycles, she had only returned to Capgras syndrome a few weeks after having enjoyed nine months of Capgras-free existence.

Since Capgras first appeared in her 69-year-old life, she had lived with me as her primary caregiver for 19 "long good-bye" months at our home. She had enjoyed a 17 day hospital stay, an 11 day experience in a nursing home, and a 10 month residency at the assisted living facility Arden Courts with memory care specialization for Alzheimer's patients.

In these two years and seven months we watched and walked down with her for six stages of the seven stage retrogenesis drama.

Carolyn had begun retrogenesis with the apparently innocuous minor memory problems of the phase called "mild" and suddenly could not recognize the husband of 44 years due to a delusion. After descending through Stages 1 through 4 in this mild phase of retrogenesis, Carolyn entered the moderate phase and Stage 5 when she could no longer select her own appropriate clothing for any occasion, needed 24 hour care to be safe, and "forgot" that bathing was a normal daily human function in our culture.

The developmental age ascribed to Stage 5 in the retrogenesis scale, as you may recall, is five to seven years of age.

When Carolyn entered Stage 6 at Arden Courts she exhibited inabilities to dress alone and use the toilet without assistance. She finally displayed the symptom of urinary and then fecal incontinence. These symptoms are compatible with a child of age two to five years old. "A long good-bye," indeed.

This she came to in two years and seven months! Is it any wonder why my whole narrative repeatedly refers to the themes of "decline," "the last time she did such and such…," "ladder," "scale," "descent," "going away/slipping away," "decrement," and "retrogenesis?"

These themes took over my life. They consumed me day and night even when I knew scores of relatives and dear friends loved us and even when I knew that competent caregivers watched and cared for Carolyn with exceptionally good intentions and skill 24/7.

But before December ended, Carolyn, Lisa and I had one gloriously memorable experience. Arden Courts provided, at no cost, a Christmas party for their residents like Carolyn and for all family and friends who cared to attend. The party was "dress up" and dress up was what many of us did.

The entire hub of the facility around which the four houses of Arden Courts meet takes in two large activity rooms and four hallways of considerable breadth. These hallways circle the other hub rooms of a central kitchen, beauty salon, staff recreation room, nurses station, etc. Arden Courts decorates these hallways for the party and makes festive every square inch of the two huge activity rooms. In every direction one can find an island of hors d'oeuvres or sweets of all varieties and quantities of drinks from tea, to hot cocoa, to lemonade, to hot cider, to coffee, etc. Live music vibrates with

Christmas carols or songs of the season, while costumed staff serve guests and patients.

As wide as those hallways are and as large as the activity rooms stretch out, the whole place buzzed with wall to wall throngs of revelers - all sober - at the Christmas party of 2014. There was us the entertained, the musicians, the Director herself on down to the degreed and non-degreed professionals who served during the evening. All segments of staff were there: cooks, secretaries, nursing assistants and those who clean and mop up even when no one is looking.

I had taken from Carolyn's closet at home a beautiful straight skirt for her to wear. Black and only worn once, it consisted of two faux leather panels on each side and two woolen ones in front and back. To go with it, I selected one of her elegant blouses: the Kelly green long, billowy-sleeved one with a collar made of long narrow bands of the same Kelly green patterned fabric which tie into a fashionable bow off to the side. She looked like the belle of the ball and got about as much attention all night.

Lisa and two CNA's dressed her and she came alive with a walking energy which would have worn out healthier athletes than Lisa and myself. We flanked her as she circled the hallways and the activity rooms like a race horse with adrenaline in to spare.

She ate precious little and smiled only some and, when she did, it was with a mystique of the Mona Lisa genre. Two photos of her by the wandering professional photographer show her in her black skirt and blazing Kelly green blouse: one with the Mona Lisa smile and one serious as an official portrait, both with me, her escort, in my black suit and shirt and red leather tie.

Carolyn did not talk much but kept taking herself and us to one group after another as if she were the hostess and needed to just touch every place with her slightly momentary presence because that's what hostesses do.

She never said thank you for the many warm compliments she received and not a soul held it against her.

The whole party stands out in my recollection so vividly with the Christmas spirit in the musical air: the guests and patients all dolled up like royalty, the staff graciously waiting on us to make doubly sure our tastebuds were filled with fluff or solid dinner, the beautiful warm, ever- present smiles, the compliments coming to Carolyn (all night) which she glided past innocently, and, mostly, Carolyn looking radiant without even trying to and Lisa and I just glad to be with her.

In her own way and in her own sphere of living, Carolyn enjoyed herself.

She never spoke a word about the party. Because she couldn't. Two or three-year-olds wouldn't have either.

This "long good-bye" occasioned tearful pains to flow and a search for more meaning than what meets the eye. The well wishes of friends and relatives certainly contained countless pearls of meaning as they spoke to console. The sacred silences between communal events breathed forth "new realizations [to emerge] from ancients truths."

In November 2014, I journaled two power-laden themes which had flowed amorphously in the recesses of my subconsciousness. Finally, I sat down and gave external form to these new ways of perceiving my reality.

One such theme overflowed into outward form on November 5 and one on November 11. I cite them here for how they framed my preparation for Carolyn's Stage 7, characterized as the most severe phase of retrogenesis by the authors of that conceptual framework.

On November 5, 2014, I journaled about a volcanic eruption that had just happened in Hawaii and the emotion, feeling, and thoughts triggered by that metaphor. The natural phenomenon of eruption symbolized, for me, all the transformations surrounding us as each comes and goes whether ready or not.

You know how the lava is flowing towards where men and women have carved out paths and built roads after leveling the land and put up houses with bedrooms and kitchens and bathrooms and garages (the stuff we are seeing in TV footage being directly affected by the lava flow).

And that lava flows with all its fire and heat burning any and everything which dares to be in its way to the ocean where all rivers go to cease to be rivers.

That flow will melt steel to molten lava-like-lakes if it can touch it long enough.

All of Hawaii's population, the powerful and the non-powerful alike, can only stop and look and observe the lava flowing inexorably down the sides of the volcanic cauldron from which oozes out, lava, so ever so slowly and beautifully, actually.

As it flows to that part of earth which humankind has domesticated, lava causes everything to start returning to the elements which all those elements were, for it burns to a crisp.

And the crisp turns to ashes and all humans can do is watch and observe and see nature reality run its course just like that same nature reality is doing all around us - ready or not

- but it is not as perceptible as the visible lava flow because it is all moving - did I say incrementally? - to another state even more slowly but just as actually, meaning, the "actual" is becoming another "actual" in the flow of life.

The metaphor which spoke to me from this is that Carolyn (and us) is moving to the state of "dust we are and unto dust we are all returning." Some at a more visible pace and at a faster pace, but all are transforming.

This is all reminiscent of the memorable metaphor which Carl Sandburg details for us as he recounts the "fifteen all-steel coaches" of the "limited express, one of the crack trains of the nation" and how "All the coaches shall be scrap and rust and all the men and women laughing in the diners and sleepers shall pass to ashes." All the while, he intimates, there is an awareness of the crack train's journey to Omaha and total oblivion of the journey on which life is taking every one and everything. [9]

My journaling, in this instance, highlighted for me one more way of seeing that a focus on the immediacy of Carolyn's Alzheimer's journey did not border on the superficial. I felt that I would be severely remiss to "not see" the underlying journey which backdrops where reality is taking us all.

On November 11, 2014, I suddenly saw not more, but differently. I understood, not only how nothing is standing still, but that everything, as it moves, does so because of an infinite set of prior motions and because everything moves due to the motion of everything - all cycles within cycles. I saw that Carolyn's movement is all interdependent on conditions ordained by a reality which "we

---

[9] Carl Sandburg, "Limited," In *Chicago Poems,* (New York: Henry Holt and Co., 1916), 40.

can perceive but which we cannot conceive," so I resorted to the metaphors of what it took to move my arm in my journaling:

I am learning "to see" that every action of mine, in order to succeed, needs to be accompanied by hosts of other actions on the part of the universe.

Like, to raise my hand, I need for my brain "to know" how to send signals of "raise" and it needs pathways of nerves to be functional enough to know how to "G.P.S." the signal to where the hand is which needs to be raised.

For the brain to be knowing anything, it requires an array of millions of brain cells, all in separate brain-compartments, to be alive with vitality. Just some of the necessary vitality comes by way of life-giving oxygen molecules.

Ah! But oxygen originates in verdure of the earth, so there needs to be in place a whole entire systematic way of getting oxygen from plants and trees on the earth to travel to where brain cells are awaiting food for thought - no pun intended.

Thankfully, the Conscious Universe does have a system whereby oxygen generated by photosynthesis, calling for a sun - 93 million miles away - to produce the heat sufficient for sufficient oxygen to flow out of plants into the air and for a nasal passage to pick up that photosynthesis product and carry that raw oxygen to where a pair of lungs (my lungs, in this case) conspiring with a cardiovascular system (mine, of course) both extract the oxygen molecules and piggy-back them onto red corpuscles riding in the cardiovascular flow of my blood and it is those corpuscles with oxygen on their backs which actually touch those brain cells for them to be alive and ready to act when signals come such as the one "raise the hand." Such is the simplified version of all that needs to be in place. Notice I didn't even get into how the sun sends the heat needed for photosynthesis all those 93 million miles (and it does it in 8 minutes).

Nor did I even go into how lungs and cardiovascular system know how to interface to make the exchange of what used to be plant-life converted to oxygen.

See, too, that to truly have a picture in completion of what is required for me to raise my hand, for example, I ought to at least give lip service to just exactly what are a pair of lungs and who or what programs them in the functioning of inhaling and exhaling?

In all fairness, for completion sake, there ought to be an explanation of what constitutes what's called a cardiovascular system replete with corpuscles the color red and who or what devised the direct route which takes those corpuscles to where brain cells reside?

It wouldn't be superfluous to address where nasal passages are nor something about the fireball, the sun, 'cause all these 'things' play such an integral part every time I succeed in just raising my hand. If any of these components were missing, I could not so much as raise this hand of mine. 'nuf said.

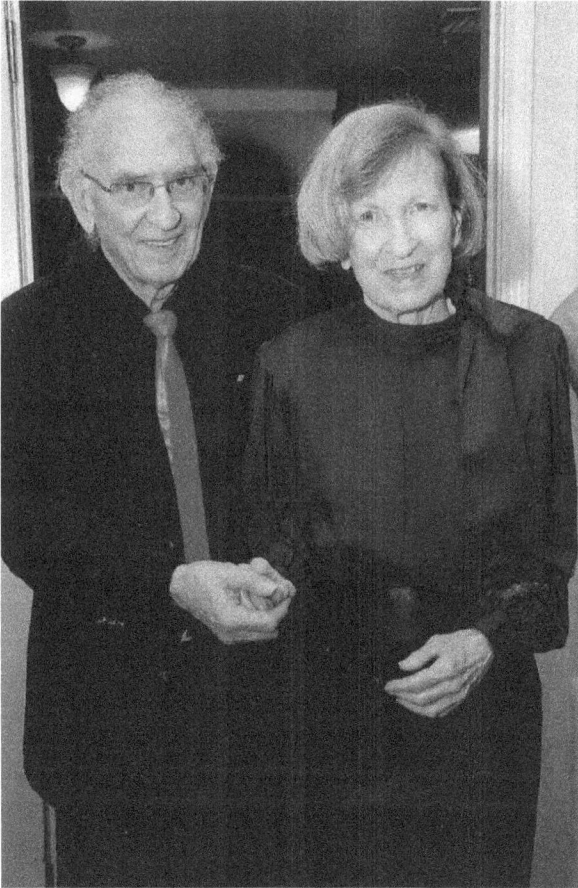

Edward and Carolyn Alderette at the Arden
Courts Christmas Party of 2014.

Edward and his wife sometime in the 1990s
Louis Christmas party of 201?

CHAPTER NINETEEN
THE BEGINNING OF THE ENDING OF THE MOMENT

The beginnings of the severe phase of Stage 7 of retrogenesis (Stage 7a, 7b, 7c, 7d, 7e, and 7f) started announcing their presence in the life of Sara Carolyn Knott Alderette and an event which had never ever happened before was about to burst into existence. Once more there was no thunderous drum-roll... no trumpets blaring... nothing announcing one of life's omnipresent transformations.

To us, it was both mind-blowing and at once one of the smoothest vortices of powerful energy ever crossed. We simply observed nature taking its course.

In a way it was like watching the river of lava flowing down to the sea unimpeded.

For months, I had been saying and reporting to others how I perceived a peacefulness and tranquility about Carolyn. As she became more cognitively impaired, I began to doubt my observation regarding what I had been calling and classifying as "her peace of mind." The doubts arose because it seemed that the less cognition anyone has, the less, it would follow, those persons can be in a peaceful state of mind. If the mind cannot function to have thoughts (which is what cognition is), I began to wonder, can it enjoy peaceful thoughts?

One of the readings to which the subject of meditation took me spoke to the heart of my growing dilemma. My dilemma was that

I did not want to be an attributing "peace" to Carolyn, if she were incapable of peaceful thinking. If her state were akin to a comatose state then that was what I needed to report to myself and to others just to be truthful.

For a long time, I did not even know how to articulate the dilemma. Perhaps, subconsciously, I did not want to even think that I was observing a comatose Carolyn or something related to that non-thinking phenomenon.

My fear was growing that maybe she was already beyond peacefulness in this life. Much to the surprise of my ego I learned that people who have experienced mystical states have been writing about subjects like peace since before formal religions took their shape and form - that has to be long ago in the purest of l-o-n-g and a-g-o. I discovered in the writings of the Franciscan Richard Rohr this insight: "When you're in your mind, you're hardly ever at peace, and when you're at peace, you're never only in your mind." [10]

"Peace," we are instructed, "comes from the heart." What vibrates from the heart is separate and distinct from what vibrates from the mind. Since that insight was imparted to me, I began to feel strongly that Carolyn would be able to experience peace even in the severe Stage 7 of retrogenesis.

By October 2014, I had been living with the reality that our Camelot had long ago ended. That euphemism for our marriage no longer existed as it used to. In journaling about this I was led to put that in the perspective that nothing was the same as it had been two years prior. That sobered me to the realization that the reason fewer and fewer out of town visitors were coming to visit was precisely because they too perceived the final stages of whatever name we

---

[10] Richard Rohr, "The Desert Fathers and Mothers: Solitude and Silence," Center for Action and Contemplation, Daily Meditation, posted Tuesday, May 5, 2015, https://cac.org/solitude-and-silence-2015-05-05/.

gave to this ongoing SAGA. Already, the increase of "life goes on" crossed minds if not lips with more frequency.

People all around demonstrated that they were regarding this retrogenesis trip as a foregone conclusion. Nobody was mean about it. On the contrary, they were there to pledge to be around after the final curtain came down. This all contributed to the experience of how the momentum was picking up. I was still not alone but I felt alone more poignantly. I, too, had to remind myself that to every end there is a beginning.

Fortunately for me, the new group of people who formed the core of ABODE, the place projected to open in December 2014, espoused a message of relationship to the now, the present, the sacrament of the moment. The volunteer training experiences for ABODE brought me in close proximity to not just their thinking, but to their way of life, their way of viewing life and death, and their way of dealing with the dying. It was positive.

The endings and beginnings which abound in our life (whether or not we are aware of them) took on added meaning from the speed of the limited express whipping us down the seven stages.

Endings and beginnings impacted me tremendously, as well as all who were close to Carolyn.

I could continue viewing her and accepting her exactly as she was: that day, in that out fit, in that mood, in that degree of awareness of her station in life, in that place. I could look at her through the lens of the sacrament of the moment.

Nothing heroic about any of this. Just looking at the trip to Omaha while at the same time I kept vigil on where we are all heading. Really! Honestly! Actually! Simply.

This constituted no resort to baseless platitudes concocted to sugarcoat the pain and suffering in life. Science has already demonstrated via quantum physics the existence of that larger journey containing all our other journeys in physical life through its demonstrations of the existence of quantum and virtual reality undergirding the physical one.

I can gather from my journaling that all of these perceptions continued increasing and multiplying. Namely, that something huge was coming to a close; that way too much no longer resembled itself!!

My realizations, I can trace in my journaling, would come and go or they would appear and I would find a way to relegate them to denial until something else happened and I would have to face the reality anew.

My gut told me: "something big is ending."

The something big was the end of Stage 6 and the reason that was huge was because of what was about to immediately begin, the beginnings of severe Stage 7, the final stage, the stage wherein the omens predicted that my Carolyn would be at the equivalent age of 15 months old!!

I did not want to dread it and yet, I did - hence the denials. (And see, when one is in denial about anything, one is not aware of it. We develop a blind spot. Denial is not a rational problem; it is a dyed in the wool emotional one.) I cannot emphasize strongly enough that what I was consciously perceiving was: "I am feeling more and more the aloneness which I have been in, since she left home especially; now I feel it more intensely."

The changes in her behavior seemed to definitely accelerate between Thanksgiving and three dates in December: December 14, December 20, and December 31.

On those three dates in December, I saw the first three evidences of fecal incontinence.

That marked two happenings of enormous consequences: the end of Stage 6 and the beginnings of the severe phase of retrogenesis in which age projection is 15 months.

The "long" good-bye was suddenly being understated.

The Christmas eve and Christmas day of 2014 that came and went were way too dim of a light to compete with the glare and burn evoked by the dreaded "15 month" age equivalency.

What I had been suspecting was confirmed by December 14, 20, and 31. Small wonder my sense of aloneness had grown to the high proportions that it had.

It is important to say out loud, once more, that what was evident to us who saw her daily, although she had now exhibited the symptoms of all of Stage 6, Carolyn was not always acting like a five to seven-year-old as might be suggested by the chart. Much less did she always behave like a three to four-year-old. We continued seeing signs of "Carolyn was still Carolyn."

The event which all these signs, omens, predictions had pointed to, from December 14 to the end of the year, collapsed into one eight-pronged seamless existential experience of multiple physical, emotional, and spiritual levels:

1. Carolyn slept all day and all night of January 4 and 5, 2015. This happened subsequent to bouts of tiredness and all out fatigue while she tried to walk. It was accompanied by the fateful evidence of more incontinence as well as a lack of appetite and a lack of desire to walk. This was so uncharacteristic of Carolyn's last 9 months at Arden Courts.

2. The Arden Courts physician concluding from testing that Carolyn was severely dehydrated with low blood pressure. But why? Extensive emergency room testing was required. She was admitted to Christus Santa Rosa ER where her records of February 2014 were housed in the special psychiatric unit that had been a pivotal part of her journey.

3. The January 7 ER visit determined admission to hospital was warranted in order to complete blood work and x-rays. Hospital sought to rule out meningitis, stroke, or other possible reasons for the new condition of round-the-clock-sleeping.

4. By January 10 all that the hospital could do was done. Rehabilitation to restore her ambulatory status had been tried and failed. All medications of a sedative type were discontinued to rule out their contribution to 24 hours-a-day sleeping. Swallow tests followed after her inability to swallow was observed, yet she was able to finally pass. (Never would have considered the feeding tube possibility mentioned. Carolyn would not allow that for me, nor me for her). Conclusion: Carolyn's new conditions were caused by Alzheimer's progressive shut down of the body. She was to return to Arden Courts.

5. After consulting with two psychiatrists, one neurologist and the M.D. on the hospital floor, I requested a hospice assessment. Vitas Hospice completed exam of all records on January 10, 2015 and found Carolyn a candidate for the palliative care of hospice.

6. Carolyn returned to Arden Courts where her room awaited her, but she was now under Vitas Hospice.

7. Carolyn's total situation was reviewed by ABODE and she was accepted as a candidate for that contemplative program for the dying. Care at ABODE was to be provided by staff and

volunteers who work with hospice staff for a person estimated to have three or less months to live.

8. Carolyn was transported, with me following, from Arden Courts to ABODE on January 12, 2015.

In all the preparations for the coming of something huge, not once did I consider Carolyn going on hospice as part of the equation. This dimension, of course, entailed a group of professionals experienced in death and dying phenomenon saying to us about our Carolyn: "We believe she has six or less months to live."

The blow of this realization outdid the giant blow of "15 months of age equivalency."

Then, in the same 24-hour period, we heard another group of professionals who deal with the spiritual aspects of death and dying say: "We believe she belongs in our program because, among other things, we believe she has three or less months to live."

This second group also studies the physical aspects of dying. I was enormously elated that ABODE, the group with which I had been training to volunteer, was willing to surround Carolyn with an abundance of love, spirituality, and genuine care befitting her needs in her "evening of life," I was simultaneously deflated that appearances were now present that by March 2014 - in three months - she might be dead.

One month prior (December 12, 2014) gave no indication to our wildest imagination what we would be asked to endure one month later. As I recalled, one month earlier, Lisa and I were barely keeping up with the belle of the ball while she reigned beautiful to behold in Kelly green and basic black. Never in our wildest imagination had we foreseen what joy we would partake in.

Carolyn had resided at Arden Courts for 10 months of her Alzheimer's journey. What that program, through its dedicated staff, did for Carolyn was outstanding from beginning to end. Two letters which I wrote about Arden Courts extol my understated thanks and love for what Carolyn received as well as what was gained by her relatives and friends.

Before we witness Carolyn's graduation to hospice and ABODE I will let my letters sent to Peggy McCarter, Director of Arden Courts and her Admissions Director Barbara, communicate my testimony:

February 11, 2015
Dear Peggy,

I will forever be most grateful to Arden Courts for the personal and professional attention paid to my wife Sara Carolyn Alderette in the 10 months she was a resident in your facility.

It is important to not only thank you but to compliment you for the exceptional environment and program which you provide for those who are Alzheimer's patients and for what you do for the caregivers as well.

I noted to the evaluators of programs like yours that what you do best is that you have covered all the bases.

You provided for the needs of Carolyn's illness on all levels. The physical layout, to begin with, was most conducive to giving my wife a sense of home and a sense of freedom as opposed to a lock-down restrictive unit.

You provided for her mental (to the extent possible) and emotional needs with programs of very stimulating and appropriate content that were delivered by a staff of degreed and non-degreed professionals attuned to real persons experiencing retrogenesis.

Your medical staff not only excel in their respective fields; it seems they represent a strong leadership to those who attend to the everyday wellbeing of the residents like my wife.

You were sensitive to Carolyn's spiritual side with attentive personnel who were (are) open to everyone's unique orientation to the life of the spirit.

Arden Courts has a wonderful host of entertainers who know how to bring joy and laughter to those who need healing and to healers themselves.

I appreciate particularly that when my wife did not avail herself of the structured activities, so many of your staff found ways to keep her engaged on other levels. I said it before and I say it again in writing that Arden Courts shows a prodigious understanding of what caregivers, like me, were and are going through and you follow through with programs of concrete guidance. Myself and six or seven other caregivers who attended a well-structured care giver program which you provided for us months ago, still meet monthly to continue the developed support and friendships begun at Arden Courts. Thank you for everything.

With respect and sincere wishes for continued success, Namaste.

Edward Alderette

Six days later I wrote to the Admissions Director of Arden Courts and sent her a copy of what I had communicated to her Executive Director.

February 17, 2015
Dear Barbara,

I would be severely remiss if I did not acknowledge and thank you a-new for the specific guidance which you gave to me at a time when I needed to be oriented and focused to be able to plan prudently and wisely for my wife's best care.

What you did for me was huge/immense/so knowledgeable when life seemed to be shutting out all the lights and I felt like soon all would be darkness and I'd be stumbling around with my wife in hand depending on a blinded man for direction. You helped turn back-on some of the lights and it wasn't long after, that Carolyn was in more and more sunlight and I knew she had protection she needed for the journey she was in.

Slowly, under your tutelage, I learned more about what you, Peggy, Dr. Cowan and the Arden Courts family know about retrogenesis and how to flow with it versus trying to reverse, stop or ignore it.

You pointed the way for what I needed to be looking for in order to provide as adequately - as one can - for a person heading towards a predictable precipice.

"I can no other answer make but thanks and thanks." (Shakespeare)

Sincerely, Ed Alderette

...and the personal touch felt like love!!

CHAPTER TWENTY
THE BLESSING OF THE MOMENT

On the day Carolyn returned from the hospital to Arden Courts, January 10, she did so in a wheelchair. She never did walk again after the failed attempts at rehabilitation in the Christus Santa Rosa hospitalization.

She acted like an awakened sleeping beauty, wheeling all around the familiar green house hallways not talking but alert. On the move she made eye contact which she knew to make in order to announce, "I am back." She was there only one day before the transport to ABODE across town.

At ABODE she was assigned the blue room - between the peach room and the green room; where her spirit still dwells with the other spirits who occupied that space for their 15 minutes of fame at ABODE.

My experience has taught me in the last 23 months of volunteering there that if a person had not yet achieved their allotted 15 minutes of fame before coming to ABODE they will definitely experience that high point of their life at ABODE.

Carolyn had had her fair share of periods of "15 minutes of fame" by as many times as she had experienced peak experiences in her lifetime of many colorful successes.

The peak experience she was about to add to her repertoire came in the form of a young woman in mid-20's who ingratiated herself for five solid months as if she and Carolyn were related as a daughter and mother are united from birth.

Carolyn, you may remember from her obituary, "had not been able to grace life's garden with progeny of her own." But Mireya, the young caregiver on the ABODE staff, became like the natural daughter whom Carolyn never gave birth to. The two merged in a union which offered Carolyn daughterly love from a source outside of her sisters and nieces. And because Mireya was there six days a week, often more than eight hours a shift, she spent that much more time caressing Carolyn with genuine loving affection than any family member could.

For the five months in which I visited Carolyn daily, I would find the two together when I arrived before lunch and then together when I left. Mireya, pushing Carolyn's wheelchair off to get her changed and ready for a post-prandial noon nap. Mireya, always smiling. Carolyn, in the hands of a loving daughter, very much at home. Mireya did for Carolyn what a nurse would have done.

By the way, just as the variable "hospice in the equation" appeared when totally unexpected, so, too, was Carolyn finding the equivalency of a natural-born daughter (for her last five months on earth).

I had slept in Carolyn's room at the hospital for all the nights she had been there and I had witnessed the talking she did when no one else was visible to me and when she had no idea I was present because I had been off to the side on a recliner.

Those conversations in which Carolyn engaged in the middle of the night and the wee hours of the morning when she had been able to start raising her body up, from the waist on up, seemed to have brought the energy for healing. This was despite the fact that the hospital pronounced that they were not in a position to help her because, in their diagnosis, Alzheimer's visited her with a condition they could not reverse.

I say this because those a.m. conversations seemed to have increased in liveliness, passion and enthusiasm to where, by the time she was discharged, she had regained the wakefulness which had been there before the medical crisis began.

By the time she took over the blue room at ABODE, she quickly became one with the spirit of the place - peace in her heart.

The dreaded Stage 7 (severe) had begun with peace in Carolyn's heart. She derived it from the air, the atmosphere, the environment of that contemplative ABODE and the real people who work and volunteer there serving as an extension of family.

At ABODE, Carolyn was in a home. She was in the home she had yearned for on February 13, 2014, when I had taken her successively to a psychiatric unit at Christus Santa Rosa for 17 days, to a nursing home for 11 days, and finally to Arden Courts for 10 wonderful months where she was one of 64 full time residents suffering Alzheimer's, in one of 4 houses, where at least eight CNA's times three shifts, took care of the immediate needs (though, not always immediately) of the 64, plus 24 hour nurses, an in-house physician and psychiatrist assisted by cooks, administrative staff and maintenance crew who also served as groundskeepers.

At ABODE, there were in total of three bedrooms for three residents considered and treated as guests. Here, one CNA per shift, assisted by volunteers, takes care of the guest while a hospice team administered the palliative care. Guests and or their families are served at a dining room table if the guest can come to the dining room. The six to eight at meal time include the three guests and ABODE personnel.

Something like this was what she was looking for when she pleaded with me: "Take me home!"

Here are some highlights from my journal of February 5, 2015:

The peace in Carolyn's heart she is deriving from ABODE from the start.

She had been bedridden for 5 days at the recent hospitalization had come alive in her wheel chair that one day at Arden Courts and from there proceeded to ABODE to manifest the air, the atmosphere and the whole peaceful environment of that contemplative place and the people who strive to be a family extension, both paid staff and volunteers and they are that to Carolyn, a family extension.

She is eating less than she had been before her medical crisis which took her to Christus Santa Rosa. But she is not emaciated. She is feeding herself but already beginning to develop some table manners of an infant playing with food, no body fussing with her for that, rather, loving watchfulness.

Family member or staff guide her to the dining room for her meals. Frequently is being wheeled outside when weather permits. Always carefully bundled up by staff when taken outdoors.

Carolyn puts up little to no resistance to being clothed, bundled up, wheeled to various rooms or outside.

I am enjoying changing her scene by wheeling her to the quiet room and parking there where we sit in silence or small talk, she still expressing what she experiences in her reality or I guide her to one of 4 corners in the large sitting room in front of the fire place. 2 huge leather couches and two wonderfully comfortable easy chairs invite us there.

I have been seeing her 6 to 8 hours at Arden Courts and continue that here. When I get there early afternoon for evening visit I frequently find her ensconced in the red leather recliner which every guest bedroom has. She'll be bundled up, the French doors open to the fresh air, pillows on both sides and one under her knees. More often that not at least two ABODE personnel are with her, they attend to her hygiene, cut her nails, comb her hair and generally fuss over her with genuine love and nurturance. People talk up close to her frequently telling what a joy it is to be taking care of her. Actually, Carolyn has allowed only one person to trim her nails, that has been Mireya's mother Maria who travels a great distance to come to San Antonio. She too, spends many hours combing her hair, and her sister Gabi, a professional chef, also has come to cook at the ABODE kitchen for a special volunteer visits.

She is changed and cleaned frequently and always with affection and great respect. Bathing is routinely done by hospice personnel who work harmoniously with ABODE staff who look after her all those hours when hospice is not around.

We family and friends are graciously treated like family too by all ABODE staff and volunteers.

ABODE provides this 24/7 total care at no cost to the guest nor to the family. The home is supported by private donations and grants from private foundations. No municipal, nor state, nor federal funding is solicited.

In the last stages, (as shown by the chart) Alzheimer's patients are down to a catastrophic 3 to 1 word a day,

Carolyn is far from that now. She has much to say 60% of the time. The estimated 40% of silence is noticeably longer than say 2 months ago.

Her conversations cover various experiences in a reality separate from ours as I have said before. We continue listening for tone of voice and bodily language such as facial expressions in order to react to her with some acknowledgement of what she attempts to let us know.

Clean, clear, crisp sentences are frequent enough to reveal "she's still capable of surprising us with remarkable presence."

These clear expressions - brief or otherwise - always delight the listener(s) and are shared with great gusto and delight. For instance, she can be handed something and out comes a spontaneous simple softly spoken: "Thank You," or she will raise her head as a particular woman caregiver walks into her room and she greets her with an affectionate "Hi baby." She can give a clear "no" when offered something she would rather not have or when some one is interfering as she tries to deliberately spill a glass of water on a table. Like a child playing? Yeah!

Many of her clear statements are unmistakably about her former work environment and her statements indicate that she in charge or that things are not in harmony. Again, sometimes her tone of voice reflects: "All's cool and matter of fact." Also speaks as if she's at a beach environment.

She sleeps way more than she had in the last 10 months at Arden Courts where she was forever on the go with her avid walking. Her morning and afternoon naps are definitely longer.

When I wheel her to a place other than the dining room table (like to the quiet room or the fireplace sitting room with the couches,) I will park somewhere and sit up close to her where we are at eye level and in this way we pass away long periods of time- beautifully spaced for talking or for silence exchanging each other's presence. I have now seen photos of her when no family or friends have been there. She is always tranquil.

I go twice a day and am usually there to have lunch with her. At all times, the ABODE personnel have been the perfect hosts and hostesses to me and other visitors. Nine times out of ten, whoever brings her to table, places her at the head place. Lunch at ABODE is very much a family affair. Four or five or six or eight are usually there for lunch.

Recently when Carolyn's niece Emily was here from Finland with her family of 2 daughters and her husband, she was accompanied by her mom Cookie and the sister Eileen who has made many trips from Alabama. During their visit, because we numbered seven family members, Carolyn and ABODE staff made up maybe 10 or 12 at lunch, if other guests came to table the crowd grew and no one objected.

Regardless of who is there or how many Carolyn and other guests on their journey home are always attended to respectfully and amidst the family talk there is an equal share of family laughter and good cheer. For a place of such abundant tranquility, there is a surprising amount of genuine hearty laughter.

About that visit from the Finland family and the Alabama contingency: at all times of our marriage, Carolyn always looked forward with great joy particularly to visits from that side of her family, her brother's family.

As alluded to elsewhere, Carolyn's nieces became extremely attached to both Carolyn and myself and we to them. She was clearly one of their closest and favorite aunts. Plus, Carolyn's relationship with Cookie, her brother's widow, had been of the best-friend type even before she married her brother and certainly before I was even in the picture. So, under normal circumstances that visit would have evoked tremendous positive emotion from Carolyn.

They were all extremely glad, of course, to finally see her. She hardly recognized that they were related. She was just not able to emote nor to converse; she could only be her silent still self sitting in her wheel chair just looking - mostly down. The grandnieces managed to evoke from their great aunt Carolyn the faintest of a semblance of a smile.

Their visit energized me tremendously. I genuinely felt sorry they could not experience more of what they would have loved to have perceived from Carolyn.

One other out-of-town visitor in this time period, whom I would have loved to have seen Carolyn aware of, was her Berlin High School (Germany) fellow cheerleader who came to ABODE from the San Francisco area.

That fellow cheerleader and Carolyn had managed to maintain what had been a close meaningful teenage relation as Army brats once they lived apart across the ocean and all through their marriages. Carolyn had relished the periodic hook-ups which they had managed to have in recent years.

Again, under normal circumstances this visit would have been a bright bright spot in life for Carolyn. As it turned out Maggie, the friend, totally comprehended the nature of Dementia and eked out for herself a meaningful visit, in spite of Carolyn's non-responsiveness. She, too, could accept Carolyn exactly as she was right there and then.

CHAPTER TWENTY-ONE
THE RESOURCES OF THE MOMENT

By this February 2015, I had been living alone for a whole year. My adjustments proceeded relatively smoothly as a natural consequence to the balance I maintained in the various aspects of my life as an 80-year-old.

I had established a quasi-routine for work needed around my house: watering plants and grass, cleaning, vacuuming, and picking up after myself so as to keep up the beautiful order which Carolyn had always promoted for every room in our home. I wanted to preserve the energy-flow which every room in Carolyn's home was used to exuding. For that to happen I needed harmony throughout the house.

Raquel, our cleaning lady, since many years past, was coming every other week to do the thorough cleaning she had always done.

She and Carolyn had struck up a beautiful friendship. We had both become quite fond of Raquel's three kids - all of whom were born during her tenure with us. Her husband had helped us numerous times by lending, very generously, his pick-up truck and his muscle for various furniture moves of Carolyn's mom. Their help has been invaluable over the years.

On the social front, Carolyn's and my friends continued having me over for dinners and visits. During the week, at least once every two weeks, I lunched with various friends. I socialized with the ABODE staff and volunteers whom I had begun to know a full six months before Carolyn became their guest. My social contacts with them took place either at the luncheon table or in private conversations in ABODE'S quiet room. This room is a well-appointed sitting area for private conversations or conferences. It serves as a reading room or place for private or group meditations. The one large sofa and four easy lounge chairs easily sit eight people and, at times, 10.

It was in the quiet room where I met with Glee Miller, an ABODE volunteer, retired Catholic chaplain, and dear friend of Carolyn's. In her capacity as chaplain to hospice patients, Glee had seen many grieving families waste a good opportunity to prepare wisely for impending funerals because they waited until the last minute and were then disappointed that they did not plan better.

Early in Carolyn's admission to ABODE, Glee took me aside in the quiet room and there, painstakingly, quietly, and pointedly gave me the benefit of her many experiences with death and dying. She pointed out that, although Carolyn was not actively dying (not in the last stages just yet), it would be wise to prepare what I wanted in her obituary, so that when the time did come for the last stages, we, the family, would not have to hurriedly put something together which could leave out much. Her advice touched on preparing for hymns we'd want for Carolyn's funeral. She encouraged us to consider music, soloists, instruments, speakers (if more than the one eulogist), the place for the memorial, a written program for the service, pre-contacts with the desired funeral parlor, etc.

My niece, Eileen, who was the most frequent out-of-town visitor, and I began a list of things to do from everything Glee suggested. We were (and are) eternally grateful for this heads-up; we feel that the beautiful service which unfolded for Carolyn did so because we had sufficient planning time.

I found it very difficult to approach all these items, especially writing Carolyn's obituary, while she was still alive. All of those types of activities drain the emotional reservoir and scare up mixtures of emotions. In the end, all the pain was worth the tribute Carolyn received. It was befitting the love, respect, and appreciation which we wanted to demonstrate for her.

Re-gathering myself from the dozens of must-do's which I felt pulling at my time and my energy required quiet times of creativity versus productivity.

My journaling provided such an outlet as did my letter writing to individuals or groups of people who looked for updates concerning Carolyn's ongoing condition. My dabbling in art work via the medium of soft pastel chalks was also a marvelous outlet.

I didn't (and still do not) have a studio for my art work but I did not need to venture beyond my TV sitting room where, with a lap-table top, me at my sofa, music conveying me to romantic memories with Carolyn, and my chalks readily at hand, I composed mountain chains, mandalas, abstract patterns... all impressionistic more than anything else and the vast majority in colorful arrays. In this, the amateur artist in me had a wonderful outlet.

For my spiritual dimension, I had ABODE's spirit and its people, including the other guests and their families and friends, to keep me tuned into the cultivation of awareness of the present moment (the one which contains "all that is").

I had begun a new (to me) form of meditation since first I entered my fourth career, the one of psychotherapy. From a multiplicity of sources I had picked up techniques for acquiring the skill of going to an alternate state of consciousness. That introduced me to quietness and stillness - the components of a meditative state. Prior to that, this meditation for me had consisted in using biblical imaginary to augment my understanding and/or appreciation of personages in the Christian Bible. In my later analysis, I concluded that I went from meditation with a religious tone to one with a spiritual tone. They are not antagonistic, one to the other; both can co-exist in one's practice.

I had begun going to a group meditation six months before Carolyn entered ABODE (and continue going weekly to the present). That weekly event reinforced my daily private practice of being awake to the present as frequently as I can be. "To be awake for the sake of being awake" replaces: being good for a reward to follow or to avoid a punishment for doing "bad."

I found it immensely stimulating to go to galleries (just as Carolyn and I used to). I also liked to go to flea markets in order to browse and look and maybe pick up something, not because that something was needed but because "you can't beat that price."

The occasional movie at a movie theater – even with their six dollar popcorn, plus walks along the Riverwalk or the market place would put me in proximity with people just being people.

Rotating the types of restaurants I went to not only offered a variety of tastes, it opened up new places and new scenes. More stimulation at the cost of zero.

For the sake of brain plasticity (regeneration of brain cells, no less) and other physical benefits, I took advantage of a generous gym membership offered through my insurance with AARP. The invaluable nature of this physical exercise showed up in my mood, my physical stamina, by grounded-ness, my ability to release tension, etc.

On days which I did not go to the gym, I looked forward to revisiting the neighborhoods Carolyn and I had walked for at least two years preceding her illness of no return. She relished studying the landscapes and architecture of homes. The talks on our walks were about what we admired as we observed. The interest she took in the plants, the trees, the flowers, etc. added such a good dimension to our physical exercise; we probably never covered more than three or four miles in our 45-minute-to-an-hour walks.

Now, alone, I have retraced many of our frequented footprints and then I added new neighborhoods to the ones we had walked. I silently talked to the absent Carolyn about new yards which I was discovering and the new fences or clusters of bushes as well as outstanding homes. I felt so regretful that we had not ventured in these directions because I was convinced she would have been enthralled at how much more beauty, harmony, and simplicity existed within walking distance… but we never went that way!

My silent talks with her gave me the distinct feeling that I was introducing her to something of value brand new. I regretted that she was no longer ambulatory. My walks were a mixture of emotions, as were restaurants without her, and lone visits to galleries or the Mercado (the market place).

Besides the necessary grocery shopping for the few items a one-person household needs, I eventually added shopping for an additional shirt or socks or the like. Carolyn had not shopped for my personal clothing items, but she was the one who initiated my shopping for me. The new nuance was my initiation of the shopping.

It was fortuitous for me that I did have a well-rounded life on top of my full-time job as a caregiver because, through those various outlets, I was very much in touch with people on a scale wider than that of the caregiving world. In my caregiving world, I began seeing daily many subtle, intense, and frequent changes in Carolyn's life. Two journal entries capture the experience of unknown certainties.

From March 2015:

In two days, Carolyn will have been at ABODE two months. Two months ago today she went into hospice. She's been off Alzheimer's meds now these two months and, yes, it does begin to show. Carolyn has not been able to stand on her own for 2 months and 7 days. Increased problems in doing so. She reverts from the use of fork or spoon to finger eating more frequently. The eating implements become more things to play with. It is very sad to see how she now leans heavily mostly to the left like one who has a poor sense of balance and is unable to right herself up. She is bruising her left arm by doing this. I cannot begin to describe how uneasy this makes me feel for her. There are more periods of no eye contact and more downward staring. (Just staring downward), she seems to recognize former familiar faces, less and less. She has more days where she is hardly talkative at all. Her voice is weaker when she does talk. The involuntary jerking of the upper body may have increased some. They tell me that is due to morphine, it is disconcerting nevertheless.

From a second journal entry in March 2015:

There are now longer periods of time where Carolyn focuses more into blank space rather than on someone or something.

She seems appreciably less interested in food. Will eat with some enthusiasm for, maybe, 2 to 3 minutes, then begins putting the eating utensils down. She'll re-pick them up but for fewer portions of morsels with an occasional big forkful or spoonful (like a child? Yes! Like a child, sad to say).

Dessert continues holding her interest; bearing out the popular wisdom that Dementia holds on to loving sweets.

Carolyn is now less and less responsive to a change in her environment; say from dining room to fireplace room or from outdoors or indoors. (Not only less consciousness and awareness of surroundings, less thought about surroundings.) Seems like profound personal fragmentation.

[Interestingly] there continue being occasional signs of risibility. Also, some surprisingly clear fully coherent statements from time to time, like last week when I put my cheek next next to hers and I said softly: "I like being close to you." She replied - equally softly - "I have a lot of people tell that to me."

It gives me inimitable pleasure that she knows that many care and can express it to boot.

I find it worthy of note that communications from Carolyn, like that last one in which she clearly demonstrated expressions of love, became a tremendous resource for me. From her words, I drew the essence of life's energy. This gave me stamina on the otherwise enervating downward path to infancy.

I literally experienced the wisdom of the social work profession's principle that, in a crisis, a small force can pack a tremendous power be that force positive or negative, depending on its nature.

Around this same period of time, in March or April of 2015, two other communications from Carolyn proved to be powerful powerhouses of resourcefulness for me. One was a remark casually made to John, an ABODE caretaker. As I was stepping out of the Blue Room where she was sitting in bed, she motioned with her head towards my direction and said to John: "I love everything about that man."

I did not hear that statement of love when she made it. John told me later, and, when he did, that small force of six words served as tremendously powerful life-giving energy for me. I felt it - and still do - from the bottom of my heart to the core of my being.

Some time later, as I passed behind Carolyn on my way to the kitchen while she sat at the lunch table with her friend and ABODE volunteer, Glee, she motioned towards me and said, "He's the best decision I ever made."

Once more, I did not personally hear Carolyn's remark from her own lips, but it vibrated all through my being with tremendous love when Glee reported it to me.

I can honestly say that my memories of these two statements of love and the total environment from which they came are resonant with meaning and they continue to move me to this day.

CHAPTER TWENTY-TWO
THE CRISIS WITHIN THE CRISIS OF THE MOMENT

When the next major crisis descended on me, a community of people surrounded me - the same community suggested by all those involvements I have been alluding to.

This crisis affected my own physical health directly and it occurred when Carolyn had been in hospice and at ABODE barely two months and eight days.

On March 20, 2015, I landed in Methodist Hospital ER with a total paralysis from my waist on down. Total. I had no use of my lower limbs, neither my feet not my legs, neither my bladder nor my bowels.

As it turned out this medical crisis unfolded in three stages! On Monday, March 16, on Wednesday, March 18, and on Thursday, March 19.

On that Monday, I had walked from my front door, heading towards the newly discovered direction of homes. After walking, maybe, the equivalent of half of football field (50 yards), I felt a strange and strong sensation from the top of my hips to barely the bottom of the hips. It stopped momentarily and I experienced what I had never encountered inside of my body - a deadening sensation. Like in one instant alone I felt no feelings in my hips. Just as instantly, that sensation disappeared as quickly as it had appeared.

This all totally alarmed my heart and my head. With that deadening feeling there occurred a distinct feel that my legs were too heavy to lift even one at a time.

I remind you, that because I had practiced as a behaviorist who specialized in the treatment of anxiety, anticipatory anxiety, panic, attacks of panic and anxiety, etc. I was highly sensitive to bodily sensations associated with "fight or flight" syndrome.

Instantly, I knew I had had a "fight or flight moment" stemming directly from the w-e-i-r-d bodily sensations (messages) at the hips and the momentarily heavy legs.

I centered myself knowing within me that the negative endogenous sensations (the strangeness) were gone, but my body's alarm was telling me, "It's a good thing you carry a cane to ward off dangerous animals; be prepared to use it as a brace as you immediately walk back very slowly and guardedly back home." That was my self-talk.

All of this transpired in maybe three picoseconds.

I walked home; I was fine but in a quandary. "What was that all about?" I was asking myself, expecting no ready answer.

The time was approximately 7:30 a.m. I took two ibuprofen - with no research data to support why I felt two ibuprofen would work; I lay down, continuing my centering by simply, consciously releasing physical tension and paying attention to the attendant relaxing and calming feelings. I stayed on the bed fully clothed for a restful 20 minutes.

In 20 minutes I arose slowly and checked with awareness my sense of balance and my strength in my hips and my legs; my heart rate and my breathing all felt good. I diagnosed myself: Alright and ready to go.

I didn't do my walk that morning. I had my simple breakfast and coffee. I showered, read some of the paper, and went to ABODE to see Carolyn.

All day Monday and Tuesday passed without incident. On Wednesday, March 18, I was in my garage that morning just rearranging stuff - no big deal, no heavy lifting, nothing out of the ordinary - when I went to pick up something from the floor. My phone - Carolyn's mobile phone - fell out of my shirt pocket and it came apart in three pieces.

Just as I had picked up the third and final piece, my legs collapsed within me. They went useless. The weird sensations of Monday returned, but this time they stayed. In one fell swoop, I was unable to stand much less walk. The heavy legs I had momentarily felt on Monday were now feeling like they were solid cast iron. I could not move a thing below my waist: not my toes, not my feet, not my knees; nothing.

The self-talk to which I have alluded and which top athletes and consummate warriors use went into double time within me and the quickest reaction I instinctively knew to take was: "Go to where you can lean up against a doorway to assemble the phone and call 911." I crawled using my elbows on the garage's cement floor. Having about half of the garage to cover since I was right about at the middle when the paralysis struck from out of no where, I was consciously thanking my Higher Power that, at least, I had a phone with me. Now, I needed to piece it together.

Continuing my slow, deep breathing and staying centered, I called 911 and requested an ambulance to transport me to an emergency unit. I had the technicians lock up my house and take me to the same ER to which I had taken Carolyn. That had been just two months and days prior.

I was feeling so incredibly fortunate that my niece, Eileen, was scheduled to arrive in two days. She would soon be here to help sort out my medical condition, whatever the doctor was going to diagnose. More importantly she would be added family in town to lookout for Carolyn should my condition be more permanent than temporary. I had already been most thankful to the Creator that Carolyn's residence was in a place of such love, care, compassion, and contemplativeness. Her care and safety thrived, I sincerely felt, regardless of my presence or condition.

I was so pleased with the care she had received at Arden Courts that I was already "sure" that that would be her permanent home until she went through all of retrogenesis. Never did I imagine that she could have even better love and affection such as I had witnessed her have at ABODE for the last two months and days.

The awareness within me put my medical crisis in sharp contrast with my multiple blessings.

At the ER they, of course, did all the routine: a vitals check, x-ray, +1000 questions. Everyone was professional and personable, from the ER physician, to the nurses, to their assistants and technicians. They could administer no treatment because none of their testing revealed what had caused the sudden immobility of the lower part of my entire body. All they could do was observe me to determine if I even needed to be admitted to a room.

I had arrived at approximately 11:00 a.m. By 4:00 p.m., my feelings and bodily sensations began to slowly come alive again. By 8:00 p.m., I had full use of my lower body once more.

The mystery just grew from no explanation for the paralysis to no explanation for its disappearance.

I was walking without crutches, without wheelchair or walker, and more importantly without pain.

The discharging doctor gave me his written report and copy of the X-ray with strict recommendation to immediately take these to my primary physician for him to determine what further testing he might choose to approach the mystery.

A friend of mine, Craig, came to pick me up and offered for me to come to their home at least for the night. I thanked him but I felt recovered. I knew I would be okay at my home so I declined his kind offer.

I was fine that evening. I went to sleep comfortably, made my necessary calls to family, awoke refreshed, had my breakfast, and called my primary's office to give a summary over-the-phone report. I promised to write up my oral report to accompany the hospital's report and to drop it all off at the physician's office on my way to ABODE. I had not seen Carolyn since Tuesday and it was now Thursday.

I printed longhand (old school) my narrative of the Monday and Wednesday episodes and dropped it off on my way to getting the prescription which the hospital had given for anti-anxiety. I had it filled, just in case...

I drove to ABODE and found Carolyn outside the French doors leading to the porch in front of her room. Accompanying her were at least three ABODE personnel chatting away, she at the center of jovial loving attention.

Suddenly, right after I had pulled up a wooden chair next to Carolyn's wheelchair, my right leg kicked up of its own volition and I felt my torso thrust back against my chair. A horrendous pain shot through my legs and the right foot began an uncontrollable shaking -

what I later found out to be spasms. Right there and then, total paralysis gripped the entire lower portion of my body from the waist on down to the tips of my toes. It was exactly what had happened Wednesday in my garage, except with a pain which I had not known and spasms which frightened me enormously and all the way down to feet and toes.

Two of the women attending Carolyn who witnessed the whole event were retired nurses. They were quick to help me keep my focus on my breathing as they applied a wet towel to my face and forehead.

I told them of the unopened anti-anxiety Rx in the front seat of my car. They quickly had me take one. One immediately got my primary's office on the phone for me. The others removed me from where Carolyn was to shield her from the alarm.

Carolyn also witnessed the whole event and never comprehended it as an emergency.

After reporting my present crisis and having had time to read the narrative which I had left for him perhaps 40 minutes earlier, my primary called back to tell me that he could squeeze me in his full calendar and that I needed to be there by 3:00 p.m. that day.

By then, I had already been placed in a borrowed wheelchair and given my one anti-anxiety pill plus whatever I needed by way of refreshing drink. I received great care and was assured they would all take care of Carolyn. Someone volunteered to take me to my doctor's appointment.

When my primary, Doctor Kayser, saw me and heard what I had to add to the written reports and the information which I had conveyed to his nurse, he prescribed steroids to begin that evening for seven straight days.

He told me that he would need a more extensive review of my situation, especially after I had taken steroids twice, so he gave me an appointment for the following day at the start of his already full schedule. He made sure that my driver understood that I needed to be taken to a pharmacy immediately in order to start the steroids as soon as possible.

My driver was the young woman whom I have mentioned bonded with Carolyn like a natural daughter. She was assistant to the ABODE Director and offered to drive me although her shift ended a full hour before my appointment. I must have cost Mireya five hours of her free time that day to drive me to the doctor's, pull my wheelchair into the trunk of the car, wait for me, drive me to a pharmacy to drop off my Rx of steroids, and return me to ABODE. Of course, every time I got in her car or out, she served as my crutch while she loaded and unloaded my borrowed wheelchair.

The director of ABODE, Jane Marie, invited me to stay in the empty bedroom adjacent to Carolyn's. Without that act of supreme kindness, I would have had to take a cab home, pay a cab driver to load and unload my wheelchair and call another cab in the morning for my 8:00 a.m. appointment with Dr. Kayser. Maneuvering at home alone in and out of bed, shower, kitchen etc, etc. would have been a super obstacle course. I have no idea how I would have negotiated any of it.

At ABODE, they put me into the bed, literally. John, an ABODE staffer, personally changed me after I soiled myself due to being urinary retentive. Another volunteer went to the closest Walmart to buy me a pair of gym trousers and two t-shirts. That was Peggy. John's daughter, Anim, also an ABODE volunteer, helped her father help me into bed for a protected sleep.

All this while, since my drama began that morning, Carolyn's care went uninterrupted. I knew it would have had I died instead of just becoming paralyzed from the waist on down. It did not escape me that I might become a fatality before Carolyn.

Earlier that evening, I was parked in my wheelchair next to Carolyn in her wheelchair at the ABODE dining room table for supper. (And people wonder why I volunteered six days a week, five hours daily, for all of 2016 and for two months in 2017. My volunteer commitment since then and to the present has been four times a week in order that I might have the disciplined time to write this narrative which I have been doing for 10 months).

On Friday, March 20, I awoke and had a cup of coffee in the ABODE dining room before being driven by Lee Ann, an ABODE caregiver, to my 8:00 a.m. appointment with my primary. The paralysis had not left, even though I had now had two doses of steroids. The first thing my primary asked: had I begun my steroid treatment the night before and had I had my second dose that morning, as he had prescribed? With my response in the affirmative he expressed surprise to see me still in a wheelchair and still immobile. This lack of change on my part persuaded him there and then to hospitalize me immediately. He explained to me that he needed me to be seen by various specialists who were going to have to order certain tests before they rendered their diagnosis. He explained further that all this had a better shot at success were I to be in one place where he could direct all these specialists to come see me and in a place where all their tests could be addressed immediately.

Accordingly his office arranged an ER and had my driver take me there immediately. He would see me shortly and make the necessary arrangements. Due to my urinary retentive condition, he ordered an immediate catheter upon my arrival to relieve my bursting and most painful bladder.

Upon arrival at the ER that was within minutes from his office, I had to stay on a gurney in a hallway for over three hours due to their backed up emergencies who were also on gurneys awaiting ER rooms to vacate. A search went out for a catheter kit to attend to my bursting bladder. The search extended from the ER inventory, to the first floor, to the second floor, and then to all over the hospital. There was not a kit to be found in that entire major hospital of a metropolitan area. Nowhere. I had never (literally) experienced such excruciating agony. Finally, a relief came when they brought the kit from I never found out from where; it felt like it must have come from heaven.

In due time arrangements were initiated to admit to me to I.C.U. where I went for the preliminary testing. I was there for three days of uncertainty.

On March 20, little did I or anyone else suspect that I would be hospitalized that day and would be in I.C.U.

A source of tremendous consolation was the knowledge that our faithful niece from Montgomery, Alabama, was scheduled to come to see Carolyn, me, and Lisa and her ABODE family that same day.

In prior visits Eileen had not only familiarized herself with the workings of ABODE, she had become one of those family members to cook in the ABODE kitchen for her family and the ABODE family of staff and volunteers and she had done it more than once.

The ABODE family that had mobilized itself to pull me through this medical crisis, while simultaneously taking care of Carolyn's approaching last days, was equally glad Eileen would be here as an important liaison between them and Carolyn's family which included a severely impaired me.

On March 22, 2015, I journaled:

I came to Methodist Hospital 03/20/15 approximately at 9 a.m. from Dr. Kayser's office from ABODE with Lee Ann driving me (and loading and unloading my wheelchair).

I have not seen Carolyn for 4 days and I really miss seeing her... longest ever of not seeing her since Feb 13, 2014 hospitalization at Christus behavioral... Psych. Unit. (My journaling goes on to report all the places she has been to and the dates and lengths of stays in various places. Like it was necessary to list all of this for eyes to see should I go silent in this I.C.U.)

To have been with her all this time highlights how strange and difficult has to have been not seeing her or touching her - Friday, Saturday, Sunday and Monday.

Today I saw Carolyn on Mireya's and Bernadette's cell phone. I would not let them show her via Skype how I look... me who looks like a disheveled patient. She is used to seeing me look well kempt. I'm looking ill-kempt by comparison, when someone can help me look presentable I want to do the Skyping thing.

Since March 18th I have now been to two ER's, two visits to my primary's office, two MRI's one MRA, one angiogram, 3 days of I.C.U.; have been seen daily by a neurologist, a neurosurgeon, my vascular surgeon, my primary - or one of their representatives.

On some days the neurosurgeon checked on me twice or 3 times and reps for the neurologist saw me twice.

I have been evaluated for Rehab. My primary tells me that after 4 or 5 days in a hospital room (out of I.C.U.) I am to go to a rehab hospital for maybe 7 to 10 days until I am ready to live alone again.

If I live 31 more days, I will be 81 years old and a day, exactly from today. "Savor the moment with all its imperfections," comes to mind.

I remind myself of this aphorism because up to now with all the testing and all the consults, my medical team working with my primary who assembled the team still has not narrowed down why what happened, happened. They witness the partial paralysis. But cannot account for it; so they do not know whether it is temporary or whether it can be spread to my upper body. Nor can they tell whether, if restored to health, this will all happen again.

I stay intent to focus on the present, the, now.

On March 25, 2015, I journaled:

Quite a trip since 3/20/15. Now I am ready to ship out to a rehab hospital. An added MRI to capture something not sought out in the others has been administered plus a spinal tap. My primary had resisted the need for a spinal tap. Consensus appears to have been that was the only sure way to rule out cancer cells in my blood stream.

Two possible causes for the paralysis: 1. Transverse Myelitis, 2. Plaque peeling off the aorta going down the spinal column and sealing off blood flow from arteries and capillaries which feed my whole lower body.

The spinal tap was negative, thanks to the Creator.

The goal of Rehab is to put me back in shape for me to live on my own and carry on as Carolyn's primary caregiver of love and protection. She has many caregivers thankfully. My role is that of the spouse. I need mobility.

In 10 to 14 days, I plan to gain strength to drive, to walk, to live alone again as I had been doing for 1 year and 1 month in my own home. To do my taxes. Have requested an extension through our C.P.A. which has been granted.

I want to resume my vigilance over my wife's care at ABODE. I am so grateful to have ABODE. Besides my physical rehabilitation which I will devote near 100% attention to so that my immune system harnesses all the systems of my body to get well, I plan to stay improving my spiritual, emotional, and mental life for all those forces which the Creator has placed inside of me to unfold and yield life for me and for the people I love and who love us.

These people are ones who have been confronted with their own mortality or just the fragility of life and did so phenomenologically. Together we have experienced what huge immense galactic force love really is, everything else is secondary.

From my journal of March 30, 2015:

(In Rehab) I am having to retrain muscles, tendons and primarily nerves and their pathways. The re-training is painful. The trainers are excellent.

The stroke has left spasm pain, dull pain, and neuropathic pain.

The spasm pain is largely gone, except at night when feet go into a certain position. The trick is to change the position quickly. The dull pain comes and goes, at will (certainly not mine), the neuropathic pain is being tamed by the Neurontin doses.

The limitation imposed by the inability to walk is a major hurdle to overcome on an ongoing basis.

At this stage of my treatments, I am well aware that just as Carolyn is surrounded (literally) by pros of all needed varieties and by loving family and friends, so am I.

The attention, love, care, and therapy which I am receiving is having an extremely positive effect in the re-training needed for my legs and feet to "work" again in the simple act of walking.

One poignant meaning I am finding in all of this is that if life sends a landslide to wipe out the road to where you were going, find another road to get to the goals you were pursuing, period!! Either that, or start clearing the rubble.

I did not come up with that metaphor or analogy about the landslide wiping out the road to my goals flippantly or superficially. When I came down with paralysis, in the full sense of the word, just as I was embarking on Carolyn's homestretch of life on this earth and wanting to bring as much worth and value to her life as I possibly could, it literally felt like nothing short of a landslide had wiped out my capacities to go see her or touch her, much less, to provide any worth or value to her life.

The daunting challenge before me was to remove the equivalent of the side of a mountain in order to have access to just the road which took me to my goal of being there for her. It did not feel like a melodrama; "daunting" means it felt like I might not make it with her down the home stretch. I was facing a stark possibility of an impossibility.

I needed to be acutely aware that the theme rumbling around in my subconsciousness about how it was possible that I might become a fatality before Carolyn was, just that, a possibility. It was not a probability yet. There was no evidence that it was probable much less certain.

Fortunately, one of the good habits that I had cultivated during this journey we were both walking was accepting Carolyn over and over again (as I have stated before) exactly as I found her that day, at that place, in that ambience. This habit had enabled me to "see" and to "feel" the "new" something she brought to our mutual encounter instead of experiencing the loss of what she was no more. The change she brought came from the ongoing creativity of the cycle of life. The cycle of life had the power to renew and, with those renewals, I had been able to live through an infinite set of possibilities which never ever materialized.

In short, without consciously going through all of this analysis, I instinctively "fell upon" or "arrived upon" doing the same with myself. Namely, I began accepting me each day with the body I had, the mind I had, the limitations I had, and, by all means, the resources I had. I focused on the tools at my disposal.

Instinctively, I did what I needed to do for myself to receive the "new" in my new environment instead of being the victim of limitations.

It was no big genius on my part to figure out how to begin looking to clear the rubble in order to find that concrete road (ability to walk) which would take me to my goals. My goals were not paralyzed by the powerful stroke; my road to the goals was. I was discovering through realization that the road had the chance of being repaired.

The "how" to my question was in retraining muscles, tendons, nerves, and nerve passage ways. And, as noted earlier, I had excellent trainers.

CHAPTER TWENTY-THREE
THE HEALING OF THE MOMENT

The following journaling of April 12, 2015, chronicles Carolyn's descent down the retrogenesis ladder and the progress which I had made up to 23 days after my stroke.

Today is the third month since Carolyn first was admitted to the program ABODE. The program of contemplative care has enriched her life and has extended her life beyond what experts and experienced professionals in the field of death and dying believed she would live. The Creator knows what we do not. Simple as that. I have been assured by Edwin - the founder of ABODE and chairperson of its board - and by Jane Marie - the Director of ABODE - that Carolyn "is wanted" to stay beyond the 3-month time period which is the norm for residents, what a blessing on top of a blessing.

That assurance means an enormous amount of relief for us the family and friends of Carolyn. She is now and has been a family member of the ABODE family for 3 months. I can truly say "me too." I also have been adopted by the ABODE family as one of theirs and in turn have adopted them as one of mine.

Our niece, Eileen, has certainly been similarly adopted as have been Lisa, Carolyn's in-town sister as well as sister-in-law-Cookie and niece Emily and our entire family. So far, these have been the family members to visit her there.

Although she is living beyond the 3 months projected when admitted, she is showing, I believe, marked decline as would be expected of one 3 months and a day on hospice. All medication intended to slow down the progression of the disease, Alzheimer's was discontinued, of course, on the day she was declared a candidate for hospice and began participating in that program with the hospice VITAS.

VITAS has been superb in its administration of palliative care while at ABODE, which has been superlative in giving to Carolyn contemplative care.

The decline we observe includes a pronounced pattern of longer sleep time. Sleep is beginning to absorb the majority of her day. She needs that more than nourishment or socialization or anything else which this life has to offer. When she no longer needs even sleep, to me, signals when the "evening of her life" reaches the midnight of her life. That is, when one life ends and another begins just as the midnight of a day means the end of that day and the immediate transition is in a metamorphous to another day.

By now "the eyes are dry, the tears are in my heart" (Say I, as I cry real tears just writing this).

I've been with her every day since she began the walk with Alzheimer's except for the last 23 days when I began my own walk with a major stroke at the base of my spinal column crippling me enough to go to an ER, to an I.C.U. to a regular hospital and finally, to where I am now, in a rehabilitation hospital retraining my feet and my legs to walk again.

Progress so far: The rehab program has retrained me to stand without support for 3 minutes, to walk with a walker maybe 250 feet without a rest, to get in and out of bed by myself, to go to the bathroom totally by myself except that my bladder sphincter is still not accepting signals from my brain, so my bladder has to be voided by someone else using an in-and-out catheter every 3 to 4 hours.

I am retrained sufficiently to be able to shower by myself in a wheel chair, of course including dressing and undressing myself from the waist on down, never had trouble with upper body. The stroke affected only the lower part of my body's muscles, tendons, nerves, etc. so I did not lose the functions of my arms, hands, neck nor shoulders.

The neuropathic pain in my feet and lower legs has been tamed to a manageable level, but inability to feel certain parts of my lower body continue to interfere with normal activities... like moving toes in the right foot, moving the whole right foot, moving some of my left foot... having abnormal sensations in the back of both thighs - especially the left thigh where a numbing goes all the way up to the left buttock. For a long time, my entire genitalia area felt non-existent.

Because of my stroke and its concomitant disabilities, I have been able to see Carolyn only two times since March 20th when my stroke arrived while I was in her presence. Fortunately, she did not comprehend what happened right in front of her.

I am on schedule to be discharged on 04/16/15 which is 5 days from today. By then, I should be able to resume independent living. I intend for physical therapy to continue at home at 3 times per week and to contract with home health care sometime soon for meals perhaps and not sure what else. The case manager here is on standby to help make these arrangements. I also have the luxury of my niece, Eileen, returning to be with me at our home for at least the first few days.

I am fully expecting to be able to safely drive my car and will welcome Eileen being with me as I take my first in vivo miles. The program here at Riosa has a way (program) to test driving ability from reaction/response time to motor skills development, to cognition etc. and to enhance needed skills.

It goes without saying that throughout my hospital and rehab days ABODE personnel who were now dear friends and truly like our extended family visited me daily and kept me abreast of Carolyn's condition and situation. I in turn reported to our out of town friends and relations the essence of what is in the journaling of April 21, 2015. I reported to them five days before I exited rehab.

By then my two rehab doctors who worked in consultation with my primary were fairly convinced that it had been a stroke of the lower body caused by plaque peeling off my aorta and sealing off blood flow to arteries and capillaries feeding my whole lower body. They were predicting that my upper body would remain untouched. They were correct.

The amount of progress I had made astounded the medical and rehab team and myself included. It all went down as if in one quick minute: a major crisis overpowered me and, in the next moment, it felt like things were already going back to normal. Just a matter of time. And the not-to-be-overlooked-genius of a medical team assembled by my primary, Dr. Kayser, who knew what questions to ask in order to get the answers needed to solve the mystery my body had presented.

I did manage to make sufficient progress to be able to go home before my April 22 birthday when I turned 81. Note well: 10 days before (only), I was bragging that I could stand up for three minutes without having to hold on to anything. (Eileen had texted Dr. Kayser a photo of me with arms outstretched in front of my walker. I looked like Moses parting the Red Sea).

And yes, our niece Eileen had returned from Alabama once more to help me make the transition home. Without her, I would have had to rely on professionals and para-professionals who deliver home healthcare - like Carolyn used to do before she found her calling in administration.

In between Eileen's visits close friends (all related to ABODE) looked after my house, brought my mail, took my laundry to wash and return, and, in general, kept me connected to the bigger world as well as to Carolyn.

When I did go home and, after Eileen returned to her home, I made arrangements with ABODE friends to pick me up three to four times a week to go see my wife until I was able to start driving again.

I felt eternally grateful to the many who volunteered to shuttle me back and forth to ABODE for me to see and be with Carolyn.

I used a four-wheel walker to get around my home and at ABODE. Since I wanted to stay my customary three to four hours visiting, I needed to have one person take me and another to return me home three or four hours later. At three times a week this employed the volunteer time of six drivers. For that reason, I did not go daily nor more than once a day. Those six people displayed an enormous amount of time and energy in such a generous, loving, giving kindness.

I continued the planned rehab three times a week at home. A rehab nurse worked with me as I learned how to catheterize myself, teaching me how to retrain my bladder sphincter so that I could void naturally.

It was April 16 when I left rehab. Eileen stayed with me five days in order that I could make the transition and to start seeing Carolyn again.

Exactly one month later, on May 16, I was able to begin driving myself. Now I could resume my twice-a-day visitations to be with Carolyn.

When I left rehab, many asked me what I had been asking myself, namely, "By when will 'they' let [me] start driving?" I had no idea "when" or "who" it would be to "let me" drive again. I simply fell into the assumption that it would be my primary who would give me the cue that I was driver material once more.

One Saturday afternoon I gave myself a relaxation much like I had done for hundreds - maybe thousands of times for patients - over the course of my psychotherapy practice. In those relaxation experiences, I had my patients visit in their imagination the performance of some act which, in a normal waking state of mind, was causing enough anxiety (fear) that they shied away from that performance at some heavy negative consequence. But, if I succeeded in enabling them to imagine themselves doing the performance while their body was relaxed and their mind in an altered state of consciousness (like when we are in a day dream), why, then they were ready to try that performance in their in vivo life! (And they were ready to try because they had had the experience of doing it in their imagination!)

In my relaxed and altered state of consciousness I imagined myself driving, taking into account all the weird and/or painful sensations which still resided in my legs, feet, and toes. With all these bodily sensations, I was still able to imagine me doing what a driver needs to do to drive successfully and safely.

I then brought myself out of my altered state of consciousness and super-relaxed state and opened my eyes with

1000% conviction that I was ready to try driving. Just to be prudent, I would do it in baby steps i.e., around one or two blocks in my neighborhood before venturing into highways and byways of heavier traffic.

I climbed into my car - a Nissan Maxima - and took on the neighborhood. In two blocks I "knew" from the "feel of the wheel" that I could do the highway system safely. I did do that and was on my way to twice-a-day visitations with my Carolyn. Been driving ever since.

I was as ecstatic as the adolescent I had been at age 16 when I first soloed.

On another front, the bladder training was succeeding with the baby-steps with which my rehab coach was guiding me.

I thought to myself: just like the entire universe is composed of would-be legos, so too, all performances must begin with baby-steps. Back to the principle: "new realizations from ancient truths."

CHAPTER TWENTY-FOUR
THE SUNSET OF THE MOMENT

Caretakers at ABODE detected signs that Carolyn registered some acknowledgement that I had returned to my routine of frequent visits. I did not detect the change they saw between my absence and my appearance in her presence.

Things were a bit different; she was less amenable for me to wheel her to the outside or to various rooms indoors. Now I would find her, if not in the bed, nicely wrapped in warm clothes sitting with pillow on all sides in the red leather chair where she could doze on and off with ease.

I will let my journaling of May 15, recorded one day before I began to drive again, give you an update:

I see decline that is visible even to the untrained eye in my wife as she enters her 5th month on hospice and, thereby, on her 5th month without the Alzheimer's medications which are intended to slow down the progression of the disease.

She sleeps (many) hours of the day indicating that she needs that more than food or socialization, or entertainment or any of our world's sounds and sights. None of us need to take this personally but she has less need of our company.

When awake, she has fewer words to say to any of us than she used to. This is not to say that she no longer has talkative days. She does but they are fewer and shorter by my recounting. I qualify that "by my accounting," because I see her only 3 times a week versus my customary 14 times weekly which I was doing before my stroke... others who see her on a daily basis witness more talkative days than what I am finding. When awake, there is far less eye contact on her part. Her visual focus frequently indicates that she has no awareness of someone's presence right in font or to the right or to the left of her.

95% of the time her mood is a positive one, mostly calmness... rarely anxiousness... sometimes restlessness to a mild degree. Instead of going into a blank stare, she now closes her eyes.

People around her continue showering her with genuine affection and attention. She still sits at the head of the table for meals... lunch frequently serves 8 people. Someone invariably declares that she is queen of the place and invariably everyone agrees.

It is so wonderful to witness the constant care she receives. So even in serious decline there continues the flow of solid good positive energy all around her and from her as well.

She is looking thinner (considerably) and that goes with the smaller food intake. Strangely enough she continues feeding herself. Although she will allow a morsel of food to be fed to her but only by someone of her acquaintance- not just anybody, and then only one or two morsels... she continues favoring desserts, especially if chocolate is in the recipe.

She used to be able to register a response at the mention of a familiar persons name- not anymore. Her expression remains the same after the mention as before. She does look for a response to the "events" which she is expressing. She will look to see if the listener shows some sign of recognition to what she just "verbalized..." as stated earlier, she can never repeat what she "verbalized" should someone ask her to repeat that.

On the other hand, she is still capable of answering when one says, for instance, in relation to a particular food: 'wasn't that good?' and she, at times shoots back, "that was wonderful." Or one may ask: "Are you hungry?" and she'll respond, clear as a bell: "I am starving." When provoked, she can also cuss-clear as a bell! Like the time I surprised her and gave her a peck on the lips, she pushed back against her wheel chair and exclaimed: "God dammit! What's your problem!" (sic)

A strange paradox is going on. In many ways, she is not the Carolyn we knew as recently as 5 months ago, and then again at times, she pops into the same consciousness which we are still in. I had no answer for "God-dammit. What's your problem?" She owned that moment. Everyone who heard her just roared.

Naturally, when changes occur rapidly, as they can while retrogenesis is in full session in someone's life, that is when one realizes that change is all pervasive and omnipresent. Normally, it appears that change is so incremental that it is not perceptible to the senses of the body. We call it incremental precisely because it is only in seeing the change speeded up (like with a time-lapse camera) that we actually see that change was taking place all along and all of the time.

In my life with Carolyn, I now perceived not only the rapidity in the change in her condition, but I experienced the horrendous rapidity of all that transpired within me since the stroke visited me that March day while I visited Carolyn. From many "heres" to many "theres," all this movement brought with it, of course, the urgent need for quick adjustment of major proportions. Fortunately, the Creator's generosity of resources (human, material, psychic, spiritual) came through to enable us, Carolyn's caregivers, to effectuate those needed adjustments to the newness of what now "was" and to the absence of what was left behind in the transference from "heres" to "theres."

The major bullet that just missed me: I was not permanently disabled. I did remain partially disabled, but a four-wheel walker and/or a cane constituted the crutch needed to get around and still attend to Carolyn. I had no qualms acknowledging that the great majority of her needs were in the able hands of ABODE and VITAS.

We, the family and friends, were in awe as to how much Carolyn continued receiving. My wet tears were now some of the times from gratitude that so many loved her in so many ways.

To this day - two years and seven months later - I will not stop saying and showing "thank you" for that kindness, generosity, and compassion rendered with love and tremendous respect.

The following journal entry of May 28, 2015, gives you up close what and how we experienced her days before the final ones:

> *For 6 days now (from Saturday to Thursday) Carolyn has been doing what she did back in January 2015 when she was at Arden Courts and suddenly she was sleeping for 48 hours without being able to stay awake long enough to eat anything nor drink anything. That had taken her to the ER admission which resulted in her going on hospice and to ABODE.*
>
> *Now, her perpetual sleep has been going on for 6 days. In these last 6 days she has had only two bowls of soup and maybe 3 glasses of water or some other liquid.*

She can barely stay awake to open her eyes, if only momentarily. At times, she will be holding one of my fingers with all of hers and by her squeeze, I can tell she is not sleeping tho her eyes are closed. In consciousness, she is keeping her eyes shut as if she were in deep sleep but her squeeze indicates she is awake. She does not maintain that state for long before she is by all accounts back to sleep.

The caregivers working with hospice' supervision are careful to be giving her Tylenol or Motrin to take care of physical pain arising from arthritis in the left wrist and fingers of the left hand.

That left side of her body I had reported earlier has been slumping to where she was bruising here left shoulder. Now that left hand and wrist have been going into a twisted gnarled position for maybe 4 weeks. Now there is no extension of the hand and never anymore of the fingers. They just won't straighten out.

She's looking more and more vulnerable and unaware of it.

Booties (technical name) have been placed at the feet due to purple heels caused by so much rubbing from a position where she is always on her back. The heels of both feet have therefore gotten excessive wear 'n tear which shows up as the affected skin turning purple. That too causes pain intended to be absorbed by the Tylenol or Motrin.

The very few words she utters now can hardly be heard due to the extreme weakness of her voice - strength of voice, just not there.

At moments of awakening she reached out to touch a nearby person or to take my glasses from my forehead to put them on the bridge of my nose where she thinks they ought to be. She does this without uttering a word. I smile and thank her and keep telling her what I've been saying all along that I love her for so many reasons and in so many ways. I don't mind if I do not get a squeeze of finger.

When she was awake enough to be spoon-fed by Mireya those two times with those two bowls of soup she was able to sit on the side of the bed one of the times and two times she opened her eyes wide-wide for a short while, soon they involuntarily closed again and she returned into another extended spell of unconsciousness.

Today, she awoke with a high fever and looked as flushed as one does when having spent too much time in the sun.

It was distressing to me to see her that beet-red. After one Ibuprofen and one-and-a-half-hours wait, her normal color returned and her fever was gone.

This evening from 6:15 p.m. to 8 p.m. when I left, she was still sound asleep as she had been since 11:30 p.m. last night. At approximately 12 noon she had managed to finish a nutritional drink with the help of a care coordinator. She fell asleep immediately thereafter.

None of the experienced people in hospice work expect these patterns to change. The rapid decline we are all seeing indicates to them a significant event which probably will accelerate.

If you refer to the retrogenesis chart, you will see that in the phase called severe 7A through 7F constitutes a person's final days of life. By this time, from May 29 on, Carolyn had gone beyond "6 words a day" and in the next nine days she would go to "one word a day" to no words a day.

She had now needed assistance to walk for over five months. She could no longer sit up without assistance for at least four weeks; she could no longer smile for at least two weeks and could no longer hold head up (like a baby can't) for two weeks. She had had no solid meal for approximately 30 days. She was sleeping the greater part of every 24 hours for about three weeks.

On June 6 her breathing changed from normal rhythm to belabored to gasping. She had been in almost non-stop 24-hour unconsciousness and, now, she was wide awake even with renewed sedating medications (to alleviate her anxiety). Her eyes were opened wide and they focused with intensity on the various people in the room including family Eileen and myself. Before this moment, those eyes stared through one's gaze in a manner most disconcerting because it felt like those eyes deliberately did not want to see the countenance before them.

My projection, obviously, because that was the feeling arising inside of me when they stared right through me. Not today. Today those eyes were strongly and intently focused eyes- like they knew or saw something we did not and could not.

A clear-as-a-bell recollection came to me of one of the training experiences I had had while we received information on the physical and spiritual signs of dying.

In that setting someone from our group asked the training hospice nurse! "And if they die with their eyes open, do we close them or do we let a relative or friend do that?"

The nurse acknowledged that that was a good question. "But," she went on to say, "that is the Hollywood version of death and dying. Our patients are generally so medicated that, by the time they reach their last breath, they are clearly in unconsciousness and, no, they do not die with their eyes open."

We chuckled at the allusion to "the Hollywood version," and I for one just took it to heart as gospel truth and dogma that hospice patients all die with their eyes fully shut. I was glad to know that. There was something comforting in knowing that.

I was looking intently at Carolyn who looked like she was intent on staying in the moment. I was struggling to stay awake to her changed breathing; awake to her wide-awake-eyes; awake to me and Eileen touching her; awake to the presence of various ABODE personnel, including Mireya who had developed a daughter-like relationship with Carolyn, and awake to the impending closing of the eyes and the cessation of her breathing.

She gulped her last gasping breath and quit breathing with her eyes wide open; eyes opened wide!! Looking at me!!!

In one pico of a nano second I realized: "I close her eyes. She can't anymore." With that, I reached over as if I had rehearsed it a thousand times and closed the eyes of my wife. In that instant I developed the belief, subconsciously, that she was so weak she didn't have strength sufficient to close her eyelids. If I had been asked to rehearse doing that I would have been extremely hard-pressed to conjure up the image as to "how to" do it.

As it turned out, my inner witness, my unifying principle, the consciousness which has been within me throughout my entire life of changes and has guided my transitions over and over again, that inner witness guided my right hand and the index and middle fingers to simply press her eyelids closed.

She was gone in that instant; she left her body behind, but her spirit, as Wayne Dyer has put it, "reclaim[ed] [its] place in the pure mystery of oneness." She died at 5:30 p.m.[11]

---

[11] Wayne W. Dyer, *Change Your Thoughts, Change Your Life: Living the Wisdom of The Tao* (New York: Hay House, Inc., 2007), 12.

The contemplative care of ABODE enables families and friends to prepare for the death of a loved one by focusing on the nature of death as a transition from this earthly home to another one. One in mystery. No amount of preparation takes away from the gravitas of this type of moment.

If I were to cite what helped me the most to pull together the many resources to help Carolyn in her journey through retrogenesis, I would quote the Sutras which I had written July 4, 2011, that had come from too many sources to be able to cite:

Sutras *

I will to accept life as life presents itself
To me - not resist, simply accept what
I am presented, in the living moment.

I will to take from life for the transient
Length of time that it gives, not attach,
Simply let go when life determines
The term is over.

I will to live what life breaths on
To me and make it what more it can be.
- Not judge, simply take it to another
possible level.

I will to stay aware and not deny the
Daily presence of the sorrowful
In life
And the transience of every solitary
Thing, event, idea and person
And I will to stay equally
Aware of the perennial flow
Of generosity of the universe

Engulfing the existence of
Each of us in the living moment.

A sutra is an intention made known to one's Higher Power.

Much later I realized: Carolyn died with her eyes open looking at me because she chose to. Weakness had nothing to do with it. Strength did.

EPILOGUE

La Puerta de la Muerte (Death's Door)
by Edward Alderette 1/3/2016

Death began opening its door
to Carolyn five months before
taking her in.

Two weeks,
one hour,
finally a few minutes,
then the final second came
one breath in, one breath out -
and she went through that portal.

I was there seeing her
ever so - incrementally, slowly
go from our room to another one.
Go from our space to another space.

Me and others there could not see
into the room and space into which she went.
The door closed quickly
and she was gone.

Her spirit vanished.
Her body was left behind.
A vacant body.
I was fortunate to be there.
She was fortunate that

others who loved her intensely
were there, too.

She did not die alone.
She did not die in her sleep;
she died wide awake.

And me and the others there
believe she was awake by choice.

She wanted to keep her silent gaze
on us - in our room -
while she backed up
into another one.
The other room.
The other space.
That's what she wanted.
That's what she did
when death's door opened for her.

Our gaze was communicating
to her gaze
how intensely much we loved her
in so many ways, for so many reasons -
when death's door opened for her.
When death's door closed behind her.

www.ingramcontent.com/pod-product-compliance
Lightning Source LLC
Chambersburg PA
CBHW070801280326
41934CB00012B/3006